CAMBRIDGE GUIDE TO
infertility management and assisted reproduction

GODWIN I. MENIRU MB BS, MMEDSCI, MFFP, MRCOG
Northeastern Ohio Universities College of Medicine

Foreword by
Professor Alvin Langer MD, FACOG

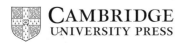

CAMBRIDGE
UNIVERSITY PRESS

PUBLISHED BY THE PRESS SYNDICATE OF THE UNIVERSITY OF CAMBRIDGE
The Pitt Building, Trumpington Street, Cambridge, United Kingdom

CAMBRIDGE UNIVERSITY PRESS
The Edinburgh Building, Cambridge CB2 2RU, UK
40 West 20th Street, New York, NY 10011-4211, USA
10 Stamford Road, Oakleigh, VIC 3166, Australia
Ruiz de Alarcón 13, 28014 Madrid, Spain
Dock House, The Waterfront, Cape Town 8001, South Africa

http://www.cambridge.org

First published 2001

Printed in the United Kingdom at the University Press, Cambridge

Typeface Minion 8.5/12pt   *System* QuarkXPress™   [SE]

A catalogue record for this book is available from the British Library

Library of Congress Cataloguing in Publication data

Meniru, Godwin I. (Godwin Ikechukwu), 1960–
Cambridge guide to infertility management and assisted reproduction / Godwin I.
Meniru ; foreword by Alvin Langer.
     p. ; cm.
Includes bibliographical references and index.
ISBN 0-521-01071-3 (pbk.)
1. Infertility. 2. Human reproductive technology. I. Title.
[DNLM: 1. Infertility–therapy. 2. Reproduction Techniques. WP 570 M545c 2001]
RC889 .M3796 2001
616.6'9206–dc21   2001025538

ISBN 0 521 01071 3 paperback

Every effort has been made in preparing this book to provide accurate and up-to-date information which is
in accord with accepted standards and practice at the time of publication. Nevertheless, the authors, editors
and publisher can make no warranties that the information contained herein is totally free from error, not
least because clinical standards are constantly changing through research and regulation. The authors, editors
and publisher therefore disclaim all liability for direct or consequential damages resulting from the use of
material contained in this book. Readers are strongly advised to pay careful attention to information provided
by the manufacturer of any drugs or equipment that they plan to use.

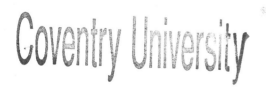

£32.95
10/01

CAMBRIDGE GUIDE TO

infertility management and assisted reproduction

This well-illustrated and timely publication provides concise yet comprehensive practical information on the modern-day approach to the diagnosis and treatment of infertility. It starts from basic principles of reproductive physiology, before moving on to the medical causes of infertility, and then describes and explains the full armoury of techniques from IVF to ICSI and even newer technologies used to treat infertility in all its manifestations. The aim throughout is to explain issues clearly, simply and directly in such a way that will be understood by doctors, scientists, nurses and other health professionals alike.

By combining basic science and medical aspects, along with 'how it is done' descriptions of techniques and medical interventions, this book offers an unsurpassed introductory account of this fast moving area and is highly suitable for the full range of personnel involved in looking after the infertile patient, including trainees in medicine and nursing, clinical embryologists, andrologists, ultrasonographers and counsellors.

Dr **Godwin Meniru**, after qualifying in medicine, has specialized and worked extensively in the area of reproductive medicine, including studies for Master of Medical Sciences degree in Assisted Reproduction Technology at Nottingham University, followed by a Fellowship in Reproductive Medicine at the London Gynaecology and Fertility Centre in London. Subsequent training and practice was undertaken in Brunei, and more recently at the Aultman Hospital in Canton, Ohio, where he is presently based. He is also the principal author of *A Handbook of Intrauterine Insemination* published by Cambridge University Press in 1997 (ISBN 0 521 58676 3).

To Maryann
for her unflinching support, love and companionship;
Chinedu, Uchenna and Chinelo for making our days full, joyful and fulfilled;
and all mothers for their unconditional love and belief in the potentials of
their children.

Contents

Preface

Many good books have been published on infertility and its treatment. However, they tend to be either very detailed and complex, being suitable for the sub-specialist or scientist in reproductive medicine, or are so simplistic that it becomes difficult to take them seriously, especially as important details are omitted. Some other books contain too much scientific material with sparse practical information. The present volume is aimed at providing adequate factual information presented in a simple format and oriented towards the acquisition of practical knowledge. It tells the reader 'how it is done' and in a logical manner.

The text is directed at a broad readership. Trainees in the medical and nursing professions, and busy medical practitioners in all specialities will find this book a comprehensive source of information on infertility and its treatment. Various professionals, such as clinicians, nurses, clinical embryologists, andrologists, ultrasonographers, counsellors and health psychologists, who care for infertile patients will find this a suitable general text on infertility. Both patients and non-patients will find this a useful source of information on matters of interest for their potential benefit or for those dear to them.

The book begins with the definition and overview of infertility followed by a brief review of the male and female reproductive systems, their origin, structure and how they function. Events leading to fertilization and early development of the embryo is covered next followed by male and female factor infertility as well as their evaluation. Some causes of infertility are amenable to medical or surgical treatment and these are described. Varieties of assisted conception treatment and their complications are considered in later chapters. In view of the expected mixed readership attempts have been made to simplify or define some scientific terms when they appear for the first time, especially in the early chapters of the book. This is preferable to listing definitions at the end of the book thereby forcing readers to interrupt their perusal of the chapter to look up the meaning. References to specific reports in the scientific literature are made in chapters where controversial issues are discussed or to support presented statistics. A recommended reading list is provided at the end of each chapter.

I wish to thank all those who gave their time to review the draft chapters for content and my colleagues internationally for their support and encouragement. I am grateful to Professor Ian L. Craft and Dr. Simon B. Fishel for some of the photographs used here. Many thanks to Professors Alvin Langer and Bryan R. Hecht for the support they have given me in this and other projects.

Where art stops and science takes over in infertility management is still a moot issue. I also realize that there are institutional as well as regional differences in the manner of evaluating and treating infertile couples. Such differences may be philosophical or historical or originate from the prevailing structure of health care delivery, funding and compensation for patient care. Hopefully, these considerations will become less important when evidence-based management protocols become more widely available.

Godwin I. Meniru
Ohio, 2001

Foreword

AIH to ZPD! A glance at the acronyms listed in the Appendix of this work reveals many terms likely to have been developed over the past two decades. During that time tremendous advances have been made in the understanding of reproductive physiology and in the ability to help couples having difficulty in initiating a pregnancy. At the beginning of that era concepts such as intracytoplasmic sperm injection, polymerase chain reaction and pre-implantation genetic diagnosis would have been considered in the realm of science fiction, whereas they have now become common and useful techniques which have aided thousands of patients. Standards of care have gone through an evolution. No longer is treatment limited to a few relatively crude techniques, but now many new drugs, procedures and microtechniques have become available to address even the most difficult of problems.

Dr. Godwin Meniru, an experienced and recognized authority in assisted reproductive technology has accepted the challenge of producing a work that will provide information as to the current state of knowledge and techniques to the various groups for whom it will be of value. In his introduction he defines the scope of the problem indicating how common it is. Changing demographics have often made the need for a solution more urgent than previously since many women have postponed childbearing to a more advanced age because of career demands and/or late marriage. Following is a well-organized work that progresses from a discussion of the basic physiology of male and female reproduction, through a list of the underlying problems and their diagnosis to a scholarly presentation of the newer techniques which were heretofore probably relatively unfamiliar to many of the readers of the work. He has attempted to present the material in an easy-to-read manner, unburdened by extremely technical scientific data so that the reader may acquire the necessary information quickly. Options, when available are discussed. A bibliography is provided at the end of each chapter for those who may wish to pursue a topic in more depth. The very important psychological aspects of infertility and its management are adequately addressed. Dr. Meniru has included the use of medications as appropriate.

Who may benefit from reading this text? Ultimately it should be the couple seeking solutions to their problem, and the work is written in a manner that allows even lay persons to gain some understanding of what is happening to them. Basic scientists will find the discussion of the microscopic anatomy and the physiology of value in their work. Medical and nursing students will have access to information offering basic understanding at their level, with a balance between basic science and clinical practice. The primary care physician, although not providing these services is often looked to by the patient for advice and needs information in order to optimally address the patient's questions and concerns. Finally those specialists working with infertility problems would be well advised to familiarize themselves with the material. Too often patients lose valuable time and resources in futile attempts at therapies destined to fail because of physicians' lack of knowledge of those techniques that may solve difficult problems and procrastination in appropriate referral to those with the necessary knowledge and skills. This book ideally should be included in the library of all practicing physicians and house officers who offer infertility services.

Alvin Langer MD, FACOG

Acknowledgements

The author would like to thank the following for their review of the text.
Dr. **Fidelis T. Akagbosu**, BSc (Hons), MB ChB, MMedSci, FWACS, MFFP, MRCOG, Consultant Gynaecologist, Bourn Hall Clinic, Cambridge (*Chapters 7 and 8*); Dr. **Peter R. Brinsden**, MB BS, FRCOG, Medical Director, Bourn Hall Clinic, Cambridge (*Chapters 11, 13 and 14*); Dr. **Vanessa Chang**, Northeastern Ohio Universities College of Medicine (*Chapters 4 and 5*); Dr. **Kylie deBoer** PhD, Senior Scientist, Sydney IVF Pty Ltd (*Chapters 13, 14 and 15*); Dr. **Steven D. Fleming** PhD, Scientific Director, Westmead Fertility Centre, Sydney (*Chapters 1, 2 and 3*); **Bryan R. Hecht** MD, FACOG, Professor of Obstetrics and Gynaecology, Director Reproductive Endocrinology, Northeastern Ohio Universities College of Medicine (*Chapters 6, 7, 12 and 14*); Mr. **Michael Henman** BSc, Senior Scientist, Sydney IVF Pty Ltd (*Chapters 8 and 9*); Dr. **Jennifer Killion**, Northeastern Ohio Universities College of Medicine (*Chapters 4 and 5*); and **Robin Whittington** RN, obstetric nurse, Aultman Hospital, Ohio (*Chapter 3*). Also, the author would like to thank Research Instruments Ltd, Penryn, Cornwall, for supplying illustrations for Figures 9.3–9.6.

Introduction

About one in six couples experience difficulty in achieving conception at some stage during their reproductive years. For some, this is temporary and pregnancy ensues spontaneously after a variable period of trying. However, there are others who can only become pregnant through medical intervention. Infertility is common, and most people will not find it hard to remember friends, relatives and/or other acquaintances with such problems. Not only is infertility common but the list of possible causes is quite extensive and to many this may initially appear intimidating. However, for conception to be possible, adequate numbers of good quality spermatozoa must be produced in the testes and delivered to the vagina at the right time in a woman's menstrual (ovarian) cycle. Conditions must be favourable for enough of these spermatozoa to ascend the female genital tract and arrive at the site of fertilization in the fallopian tube. They should be functionally adequate for the task of breaking through the cells that surround the oocyte to enable one of them to fertilize the oocyte. The fertilized egg should develop normally and implant successfully when it arrives at the uterine cavity as an embryo. Difficulty with conception will be experienced if any factor prevents the successful completion of these events.

It is estimated that 80 out of 100 couples are able to achieve pregnancy within one year of having regular sexual intercourse without contraceptives. Ten more couples will get pregnant in the second year while the remaining 10 couples are not able to do so within that time frame and are said to be infertile. However, some of these infertile couples may still achieve pregnancies without any assistance in the third or subsequent years of trying. Since it took them all this time to get pregnant they are said to be subfertile; their fertility is impaired to some extent but not completely. The remaining couples (usually 3–5%) rarely achieve conception unless some form of treatment is provided. This is because one or both members of the couple could be sterile. Infertility therefore encompasses subfertility and sterility. Infertility is defined as an inability to achieve pregnancy within two years of having regular unprotected intercourse. Some authorities may use one year as the cut-off point. Infertility is a problem of the couple. None of the partners can be said to be infertile; one or both partners may be subfertile or sterile. There are about 60–80 million infertile couples world-wide. Infertility is said to be primary if the couple have had no previous pregnancy and secondary if there has been at least one pregnancy irrespective of its outcome (miscarriage, ectopic pregnancy and preterm or term delivery). The male partner is solely responsible in 40% of infertility cases while the female partner is responsible for another 40%. Both are responsible for the remaining 20% of cases.

Steady progress has been made in recent decades in the treatment of infertility. Consequently, a large proportion of infertile couples should now have a realistic expectation of being able to have children, although it may take time and many treatment attempts for this to happen. Treatment could be by the administration of medication or performing surgery or a combination of both. Couples in whom these treatments are unsuccessful or are not suitable can have assisted conception treatment; several thousand babies have now been delivered world-wide following the birth of the first so-called 'test-tube' baby in 1978. Infertility is associated with psychological upheaval and perpetual mental anguish. Furthermore, infertility treatments impose physical, social, financial and mental stress on the couple. The stress is worse with the assisted reproduction technologies and success is not guaranteed in the first or any specific cycle of treatment. Knowledge and information are the best tools with which infertile couples can tackle their problem and obtain the best possible treatment for themselves. They need to know about their bodies and how conception takes place. They also need to know when, how and where to seek assistance for their continued inability to conceive. They should be aware of the various available treatment modalities, their efficacy and drawbacks. Their knowledge of the subject matter should be enough to allow them to follow their treatment as it progresses thereby making for better compliance with the treatment regimens. A book such as this fulfils these objectives. In addition, it ensures that the busy practitioner and the non-medical members of the team have access to a simple yet comprehensive text, that will enable them to optimally perform their various roles in the care of infertile patients.

The male reproductive system

Introduction

The anatomy and function of the male genital organs fulfil certain roles during the reproductive process; copies of the man's genetic make up are packaged in spermatozoa which are produced in the testes. These gametes are then conducted along the male genital tract. Ejaculation results in their deposition in the vagina if intravaginal intercourse takes place. A simplified physiological anatomy of the male genital tract will be presented in this chapter.

The male sex organs

The male sex organs consist of the testes, excretory ducts, accessory glands and the penis (Table 1.1 and Figure 1.1). The testes (singular: testis) are two oval structures that normally lie in the scrotum (Figure 1.2). Each testis measures 4–6 cm in length and has a volume of about 25 ml. The testes produce spermatozoa (singular: spermatozoon) and testosterone (the male hormone). A mature spermatozoon is shown in Figure 1.3. It is a highly specialized cell that is designed for movement. The sole function of the spermatozoon is to carry a copy of the man's genetic make up, in the form of chromosomes, from the site of production in the testis, through the male and female genital tracts, to the egg that it fertilizes. The spermatozoon carries this genetic material in the head piece. The rest of the spermatozoon is made up of the mid-piece, which supplies the energy, and the tail which propels the sperm forward.

Production of spermatozoa commences at puberty and takes place inside highly coiled tubes that are found in the testes called seminiferous tubules (Figure 1.4). Following their production, spermatozoa are wafted along the seminiferous tubules, by a fluid current, and enter the excretory ducts. The epididymis is a highly coiled tube measuring 5–6 m if unwound fully. It connects the tubules of the testis to the vas deferens. The vas deferens is 35–45 cm long. From its point of origin in the scrotum the course of the vas deferens is upwards to the groin. It then enters

Table 1.1. The male reproductive organs

Components	Number
Testis	2
Excretory ducts	
epididymis	2
vas deferens	2
Accessory sex glands	
seminal vesicle	2
prostate	1
bulbo-urethral gland	2
Ejaculatory duct	2
Urethra	1
Penis	1

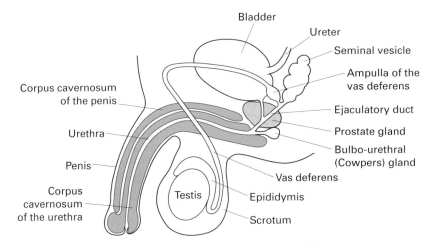

Figure 1.1   The male sex organs: side view.

the body cavity through a tunnel (called the inguinal canal) where it joins the duct of the seminal vesicle on that side to form the ejaculatory duct. Spermatozoa reaching the ejaculatory duct from the vas deferens of each side are ejected from the penis, which is the copulation organ, together with secretions from the accessory sex glands (seminal vesicles, prostate gland and bulbo-urethral glands) at the time of ejaculation. The urethra also conducts urine from the bladder to the exterior during urination. The prostate is the largest accessory sex gland. It weighs 20 g and is 3–4 cm in diameter.

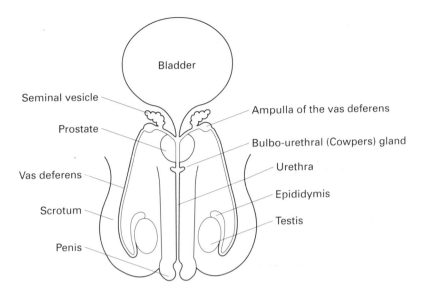

Figure 1.2   The male sex organs: front view showing paired components.

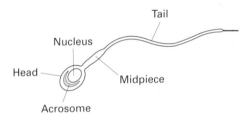

Figure 1.3   A mature spermatozoon.

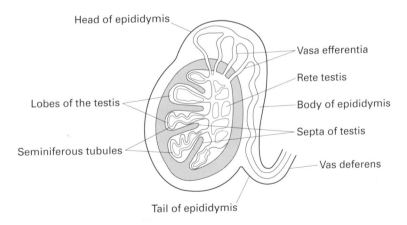

Figure 1.4   Section through the testis showing the organization of the various systems of tubules.

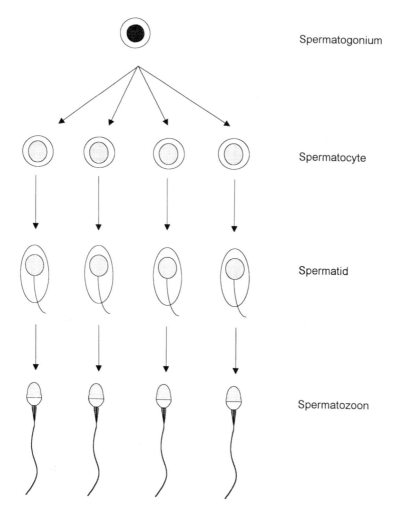

Figure 1.5   Major stages during production of spermatozoa in the testes.

Production of spermatozoa

The testes hang well out of the body cavity in the scrotum; this is necessary to keep the testes cooler than the rest of the body which is at 37 °C. The temperature of the testes while in the scrotum can be up to 4–7 °C lower than that of the body. The lower temperature is required for optimal production of spermatozoa. Spermatozoa develop from spermatogonia which are cells that line the inside of the seminiferous tubules. The spermatogonia do not just change into spermatozoa. They divide repeatedly and the resulting cells go through a complex series of changes before becoming fully formed spermatozoa (Figures 1.5 and 1.6). These processes take about 64 days to be complete in the testes. It then takes another

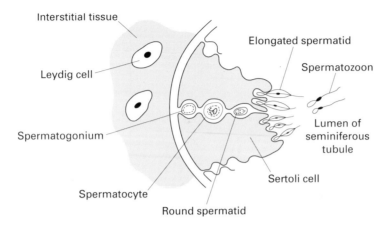

Interstitial tissue

Elongated spermatid

Spermatozoon

Leydig cell

Spermatogonium

Lumen of
seminiferous
tubule

Spermatocyte

Sertoli cell

Round spermatid

Figure 1.6   Transverse section through a seminiferous tubule and adjoining interstitial tissue.

10–14 days for these spermatozoa to pass through the epididymis and vas deferens. Although fully formed in the testes, spermatozoa are not completely mature and do not usually move. Their transit through the seminiferous tubules and into the epididymis is as a result of movement of the fluid in which they are suspended. The fluid current is set up by Sertoli cells which continuously secrete fluid into the seminiferous tubules. Sertoli cells are one of the groups of cells found within the seminiferous tubules. The spermatozoa may begin to move when they enter the epididymis but the movement tends to be in circles. Full motility is however achieved by the time they leave the epididymis. The epididymis acts as a storage organ for spermatozoa. The vas deferens also acts as a storage organ but the number of spermatozoa it contains at any point in time is usually just enough for one ejaculation. The transport of spermatozoa through the epididymis and vas deferens is by means of contraction of muscles found within the walls of these hollow tubular structures.

Development of the testis

The testes originally lie in the abdomen of the developing male fetus but descend into the scrotum during the later part of pregnancy. Cells that will eventually produce spermatozoa (called primordial germ cells) are deposited in the testes in the early stage of testicular development. These primordial germ cells arise in the yolk sac of the embryo and migrate, between the fourth and sixth week of pregnancy, to the genital ridge that eventually forms the testes. The primordial germ cells develop into spermatogonia and lie dormant until the boy reaches puberty when the spermatogonia resume cell division and further development. The testes

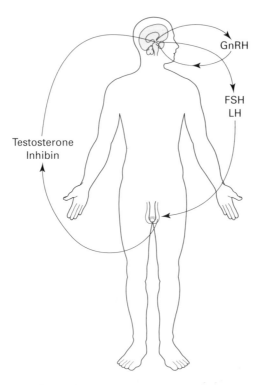

Figure 1.7   An adult male and the distance separating the hypothalamus and pituitary gland from the male sex organs.

do not become depleted of spermatogonia unlike the situation in the female, as will be seen in Chapter 2.

Hormones that control the function of the adult male sex organs

The hypothalamus and pituitary gland are located in the brain and influence the function of the male sex organs, although they themselves are not sex organs. Both glands secrete hormones (Figure 1.7). Gonadotrophin releasing hormone (GnRH) is one of the hormones secreted by the hypothalamus. GnRH enters blood vessels in the brain to reach the pituitary gland which it stimulates to produce two other hormones. One is the follicle stimulating hormone (FSH) while the other is the luteinizing hormone (LH). Both FSH and LH are secreted into the blood stream through which they reach the sex organs. Inhibin, another hormone, is produced by Sertoli cells, while testosterone is produced by cells that lie outside the seminiferous tubules – the Leydig cells. FSH stimulates the production of spermatozoa within the seminiferous tubules while LH stimulates Leydig cells to produce testosterone. FSH also contributes to the stimulation of Leydig cells to produce testosterone (Figure 1.8).

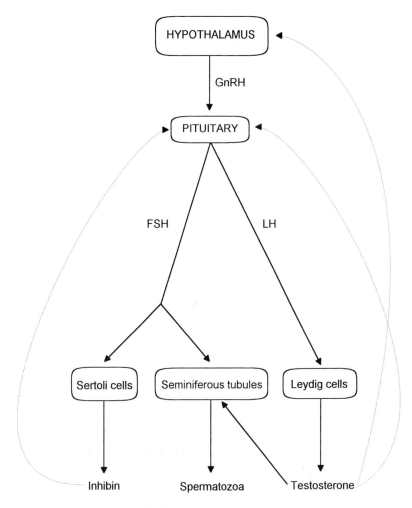

Figure 1.8   Hormonal control of testicular function.

In the adult, testosterone maintains the size and function of the various sex organs and is important for the production of spermatozoa. Feedback control mechanisms are present in various organs of the body and help to keep the production of compounds and materials at a constant level. In relation to the male reproductive organs, testosterone controls the production of LH; when the concentration of testosterone in blood decreases, the release of LH is increased and vice versa. Part of the feedback control of testosterone on LH production is through its effect on the production of GnRH by the hypothalamus. When the production of spermatozoa drops, the production of inhibin by the Sertoli cells also drops. The pituitary senses the low level of inhibin and increases the production of FSH. FSH then stimulates production of more inhibin and spermatozoa (Figure 1.8).

Table 1.2. Constituents of semen

Cells	Chemical compounds
Spermatozoa	Water
White blood cells	Hormones
Epithelial cells	Proteins
(Red blood cells)	Carbohydrates
(Bacteria)	Steroids
(Viruses)	Lipids
	Other compounds

Erection and ejaculation

Sexual arousal and excitement in men result from input of the various senses (sight, touch, sound, smell and taste). Erection of the penis is usually one of the earliest manifestations of sexual arousal. There is also erection of the nipples, increase in the heart rate and blood pressure. The excitement is maintained and even increased by sexual intercourse or masturbation. At the height of sexual excitement the smooth muscles in the walls of the epididymides and vasa deferentia (plural of vas deferens) contract and expel spermatozoa into the urethra. The muscles in and around the prostate and seminal vesicles also contract and these glands discharge their secretions into the urethra. This is also the time during which the man begins to orgasm; there is a release of sexual tension and arousal and the man has an intense feeling of pleasure. The muscles at the neck of the bladder contract and this prevents spermatozoa and the secretions from flowing back and into the bladder. Within a very short period after the emission of spermatozoa and the accessory sex gland secretions, there is repeated contraction of the muscles of the pelvis, lower extremities and the trunk. The smooth muscles of the urethra contract along with other muscles in the penis. This has the effect of expelling semen from the urethra to the outside which if the man is having vaginal sexual intercourse at that time, will be expelled into the vagina.

Composition of semen

Semen is the fluid that is ejected from the penis at the time of orgasm. It should not be confused with pre-ejaculatory fluid which is produced by the bulbo-urethral glands during sexual excitement and before ejaculation. Pre-ejaculatory fluid is thin and clear and serves to flush the urethra and neutralise any acidic remnants of urine. The constituents of semen are shown in Table 1.2. The volume of semen produced during ejaculation is usually between 2 and 6 ml. The seminal vesicles contribute about two-thirds of the fluid while the prostate contributes one-third. The contribution to this volume by fluid from the testes, via the epididymides and vasa deferentia, is negligible. The most apparent contribution of the testes to semen are spermatozoa. Normally, both live and dead spermatozoa are found in semen together with a small number of white blood cells. These white blood cells serve the function of guarding the genital tract from infection just as in other parts of the body where they are found. They tend to engulf any micro-organism (such as bacteria) they find but they also engulf dead cells, including dead spermatozoa. When the number of white blood cells found in semen is high it may mean that there is an infection in the male genital tract. However, even after extensive investigation no source of infection will be found in a large proportion of cases. Epithelial cells can also be found in semen. These are cells that cover the surface of the genital tract and it is normal to find some in semen. Debris are found in semen and represent fragments of broken down cells and other material. Occasionally red blood cells or bacteria can be found in semen. This finding is not normal and all attempts should be made to find out the exact cause of the problem and provide appropriate treatment. It is now being realized that viruses can also be found in semen and may have a role in the causation of infertility in some couples. Semen contains numerous chemical compounds produced by the accessory sex glands. These compounds have different functions including protection and nourishment of spermatozoa. The fluid also helps to transport the spermatozoa along parts of the male genital tract. Following ejaculation the fluid protects spermatozoa from the acidic conditions of the vagina long enough for some of them to escape into the upper parts of the female genital tract. Initially after ejaculation semen forms a clot due to the action of a coagulation enzyme produced by the seminal vesicles. However, the clot begins to liquefy after a few minutes due to the liquefactive activity of seminine, an enzyme produced by the prostate gland; the process is complete usually within 30 minutes.

Semen parameters

As will be seen in Chapter 6, semen is analysed during the evaluation of couples who have difficulty in achieving pregnancies. The aim of this analysis is to determine if the various constituents of semen are present and in the right proportions. Attempts have been made to define normal semen parameters. Although these attempts are continuing, the following parameters are accepted as normal for the time being. Semen should liquefy within 30–60 minutes of ejaculation. Liquefied semen is not viscous. It should have a greyish-white appearance. At times it may appear a little yellowish but this is also accepted as normal. Semen should not be clear like water, it should have a translucent appearance. It should not be acidic or too alkaline. This can be measured easily in the laboratory. The pH of semen should be 7.2 or more (i.e. neutral to slightly alkaline). The odour of semen has been described as being 'fresh'. Semen should not have an offensive odour. The volume of semen collected from one ejaculation is usually above 2 ml.

The concentration of spermatozoa in the semen sample should normally exceed 20 million spermatozoa in 1 ml of the sample. What this means is that one ejaculate may contain a total of 40 million spermatozoa if the concentration is 20 million/ml and the volume of semen is 2 ml. For an ejaculate of 6 ml with a concentration of 20 million/ml, the total number of spermatozoa will then be 120 million. Semen samples with a higher concentration will have a greater number of spermatozoa in the ejaculate. It is quite possible for a total count of 600 million spermatozoa to be found in an ejaculate. Higher values have also been recorded. At least 50% of the spermatozoa should be moving. The proportion of live spermatozoa in the sample is normally 75% or greater. A large proportion of spermatozoa are abnormal in appearance even if they are alive and moving. No one knows why this is so but this finding is universal; all men produce semen containing abnormal looking spermatozoa. However, at least 15–30% of spermatozoa in a sample should look normal. Further discussions on semen parameters can be found in Chapters 4 and 6.

Applied concepts

- It is recommended that a man should not ejaculate for a period of 2–5 days before producing a semen sample for analysis. This is an attempt to ensure that every patient coming for semen analysis has the same period of abstinence. In so doing it becomes easier to interpret the results of the analysis and compare results from different patients.
- The concentration of spermatozoa in semen and some of the other parameters do not remain constant in all semen samples produced by the same individual. The concentration, for example, varies from sample to sample. That is why it is necessary to repeat semen analysis on the same man at least three times over a period of a few months to gain a full impression of how much the concentration varies from sample to sample. This is even more important if a poor result is obtained when semen analysis is performed on a man for the first time. Having said this, a man who, for example, produces a sample that has a sperm concentration of 100 million/ml is not likely to produce a sample that has a concentration of 5 million/ml. Of course he needs to abstain from ejaculation for the standard period of time and should not have any illness or ingest any drug that will decrease the production of spermatozoa during the interval between tests.

- It takes about 74–78 days for spermatozoa to be produced and appear in the ejaculate. This means that it will take that length of time, at a minimum, to find out if a bout of illness or ingestion of toxic substances or drugs affects the production of spermatozoa. It will also take that length of time to find out if treatment has had any beneficial effect on the production and quality of spermatozoa.

- Production of semen for analysis is usually by masturbation into a special sterile plastic container supplied by the laboratory. The container is labelled with the man's name, date of birth, hospital number, date and time of production of the sample, and other identifying information. The container is closed properly after collection of semen and taken to the laboratory.

- Many laboratories ask for semen samples to be produced on site. This is to enable analysis of the sample to be commenced within a short time (about 30 minutes) of its production. The longer a sample is left before analysis the harder it is to exclude the long interval as a cause of abnormal results, particularly for the assessment of motility of the spermatozoa and the percentage that are alive. Producing the sample at the laboratory also avoids the semen being exposed to extremes of temperature conditions during transport to the laboratory.

- Special rooms are set aside at the laboratory or hospital for the production of semen samples. The room is located in a quiet part of the unit and a 'do not disturb' sign is usually hung on the door. Visual aids in the form of magazines and video tapes are provided by most establishments for men who require them.

- Men who find it difficult masturbating at the laboratory or hospital are allowed to produce the sample at home by masturbation. They are usually asked to bring in the sample to the laboratory as soon as possible, within 30 minutes and not more than one hour from the time of production.

- No lubricants are allowed to be used during masturbation. This is because most lubricants are toxic to spermatozoa and may adversely affect the results of the semen analysis if they come in contact with the semen.

- Some men may find it impossible to masturbate. They are provided with special condoms to use during normal sexual intercourse. These condoms are unlike all other condoms because they are made of materials, for example medical grade silicone rubber, that are non-toxic to spermatozoa. The normal contraceptive condoms contain chemicals that kill spermatozoa, for example, nonoxynol-9 and nonoxynol-11. Following ejaculation the condom is removed and the semen emptied into a sterile plastic container before being sent to the laboratory.

- The production of spermatozoa by the testes, hence fertility, decreases with age. However, this may not be pronounced in many men and men have fathered children well into their old age. The effect of age on fertility is more evident in females.

- When a man does not ejaculate for some time the accumulated spermatozoa in the vas deferens dribble into the urethra where they are washed away by urine. This serves to prevent a build up of pressure in the testis, epididymis and vas deferens. It however does not mean that all accumulated spermatozoa will be discharged into the urethra this way. Some will still remain in the genital tract and eventually die.
- Avoiding ejaculation for a few days may increase the number of spermatozoa in the ejaculate. Abstinence for long periods of time, however, will not lead to any more improvement of the semen quality. Instead, the number of dead sperm will increase and this may impair the overall quality of the semen sample. Abstinence for more than 3–5 days is not likely to improve the semen quality further.

BIBLIOGRAPHY

Grudzinskas, J. G. & Yovich, J. L. (Eds) (1995). *Gametes – The Spermatozoon.* Cambridge: Cambridge University Press.

Johnson, M. & Everitt, B. (2000). *Essential Reproduction,* 5th edn. London: Blackwell Science.

Knobil, E. & Neill, J. D. (Eds), Greenwald, G. S., Markert, C. L. & Pfaff, D. W. (Associate Eds) (1994). *The Physiology of Reproduction,* 2nd edn. New York: Raven Press.

Rowe, P. J., Comhaire, F. H., Hargreave, T. B. & Mahmoud, A. M. A. (2000). *WHO Manual for the Standardized Investigation, Diagnosis and Management of the Infertile Male.* Cambridge: Cambridge University Press.

Rowe, P. J., Comhaire, F. H., Hargreave, T. B. & Mellows, H. J. (1993). *WHO Manual for the Standardized Investigation and Diagnosis of the Infertile Couple.* Cambridge: Cambridge University Press.

World Health Organization (1992). *WHO Laboratory Manual for the Examination of Human Semen and Sperm-Cervical Mucus Interaction,* 3rd edn. Cambridge: Cambridge University Press.

World Health Organization (1999). *WHO Laboratory Manual for the Examination of Human Semen and Sperm-Cervical Mucus Interaction,* 4th edn. Cambridge: Cambridge University Press.

2

The female reproductive system

Introduction

The female reproductive system is made up of the sex organs and associated structures, both remote and near. The female genital tract provides an avenue for the transport of spermatozoa from their point of deposition in the vagina to the place where fertilization of the released oocyte occurs. The function of the ovaries is regulated such that one of them produces an oocyte each month. The release of the oocyte from the ovary is timed to correspond to the period when the reproductive tract is best suited for implantation if this oocyte happens to become fertilized. If fertilization and/or implantation do not occur, the changes in the reproductive tract are rapidly reversed to allow a new cycle of changes to commence. This ensures that the possibility of fertilization and implantation is always maintained in each new cycle.

The female sex organs

The female sex organs can be broadly grouped into two: the internal and external genitalia (Table 2.1 and Figures 2.1–2.3). The vulva is another name for the external genitalia. The mons pubis (or mons veneris) is the hair bearing area of skin overlying the pubic symphysis (which is the joint formed between the two pubic bones in front). Underneath the skin is a pad of fat which provides some cushioning between the pubic bones of both partners during sexual intercourse. This hair bearing skin extends backwards on either side of the vaginal introitus (vaginal opening) to become the labia majora. The labia majora are similar to the mons pubis in having underlying fatty tissue. They merge posteriorly to form the perineum (Figure 2.1). The labia minora lie on the inside of the labia majora and on each side of the vaginal introitus. They consist of two thin delicate folds of skin which vary in size amongst individuals; in some females the labia minora are prominent while in others they are relatively small and may be covered by the labia majora.

Table 2.1. The female sex organs

External genitalia	Internal genitalia
Mons veneris	Vagina
Labia majora	Uterine cervix
Labia minora	Uterine body
Clitoris	Fallopian tubes
Vaginal introitus	Ovaries
Bartholin's glands	
Hymen	
Vestibule	
External urethral meatus	

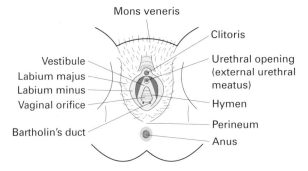

Figure 2.1   The female external genitalia.

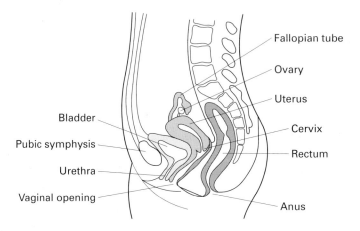

Figure 2.2   Longitudinal section through the female pelvis showing the internal genitalia and other pelvic organs.

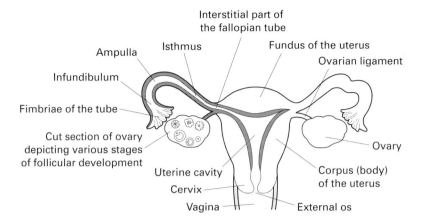

Figure 2.3   Section through the uterus, right fallopian tube and ovary.

The clitoris is the female equivalent of the penis. It has a rich nerve supply and this makes it one of the most erogenous structures in the body. The urethral opening is called the external urethral meatus and is found on the vestibule which is the triangular area of skin lying between the labia minora and the vaginal introitus. The hymen is a thin membrane found around the vaginal introitus. It is usually intact in females who have not had sexual intercourse. The first intercourse tears the hymen but there is not much bleeding because it has few blood vessels. The hymen can also be disrupted during operations on the vagina, insertion of tampons to contain menstrual bleeding or if the finger is forcibly inserted into the vagina. Childbirth destroys the hymen completely, leaving a few tags of tissue called the carunculae myrtiformes. The Bartholin's glands are the equivalent of the Cowper's glands in the male and lie behind and to the side of the vaginal introitus. They are quite small (pea sized) and normally cannot be felt. Their secretions help lubricate the vulva and vagina during sexual intercourse.

The vagina extends backwards and upwards from the vaginal introitus. The vagina is kept acidic in an attempt to prevent harmful bacteria from getting to the upper parts of the female genital tract. This acidity is caused by the action of a 'friendly' type of bacteria called Doerdelein's bacilli. These organisms are present in the vagina from puberty onwards and act on the glycogen-rich vaginal secretion converting it into lactic acid. The cervix is found at the upper portion of the vagina. The opening of the cervix seen from the vagina is called the external os (Figure 2.4) and leads into the cervical canal. The lining of the cervical canal has many infoldings (also called crypts or glands) (Figure 2.5). The cells that provide this lining secrete mucus. It is believed that the crypts of the cervix act as a reservoir for spermatozoa. The point at which the cervical canal joins the cavity of the uterus is called the internal os. The uterus is a pear shaped organ which is actually made up of two

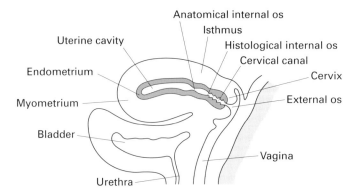

Figure 2.4   Longitudinal section through the uterus showing the anatomical landmarks of the cervix and cervical canal.

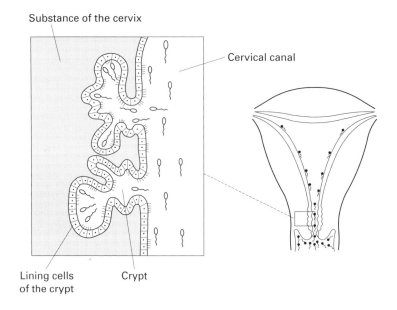

Figure 2.5   Crypts (glands) of the cervical canal.

components – the uterine body and the uterine cervix. The cervix has already been described. The uterine body is composed mainly of smooth muscle fibres called the myometrium. The overall length of the uterus is about 8–9 cm while the width, at its widest point, is 6 cm. The uterus weighs 45–55 g. Its size varies amongst individuals – it is slightly larger in females who have had previous pregnancies, and tends to be small before puberty and after the menopause. The uterine cavity is lined by the endometrium which is the layer where the embryo implants after fertilization. The myometrium is lined on the outside mainly by peritoneum.

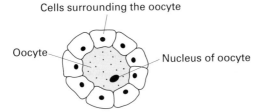

Figure 2.6   A primordial follicle consisting of an oocyte surrounded by a layer of cells.

The fallopian tubes form a conduit between the uterine cavity and ovaries. Each tube is about 10 cm long. The end of the tube flares out like a trumpet and has finger-like processes (called fimbriae) that help with the capture of the oocyte after ovulation. This end of the tube tends to hover over the ovaries at the time of ovulation. The ovaries are ovoid structures and each is about 3.5 cm long weighing 4–8 g. The ovaries produce oocytes and the female sex hormones.

Development of the ovary

The ovaries are formed in the abdomen and move slightly downwards to enter the pelvic cavity during development of the female fetus. They do not migrate further downwards, unlike the testes that move down to the scrotum in the later part of pregnancy. All oocytes a female will ever have are produced and stored in her ovaries while she is still in the womb. Each oocyte is usually surrounded by cells and this combination of the oocyte and the surrounding cells is called a follicle. The earliest developmental stage of the ovarian follicle is called the primordial follicle (Figure 2.6). Production of these primordial follicles stops before the female child is born. In fact the ovaries contain the maximum number of primordial follicles they will ever have (6 000 000) at about five months of pregnancy. From then onwards many of these follicles degenerate and are lost. The ovaries contain about 500 000 primordial follicles at birth. By puberty 250 000 remain. By the age of 25 years the ovaries contain roughly 60 000 primordial follicles and this drops to 8000 by the age of 40. A female will probably not ovulate more than 500 oocytes in her lifetime.

Ovarian cycle

Following puberty there are activities that take place in the ovaries in a cyclical manner. At intervals a group of up to 20 or more primordial follicles begin to develop further. The first noticeable change is an increase in the size and number of cells surrounding each oocyte. However, within a few days only one follicle

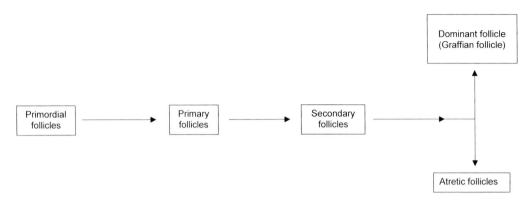

Figure 2.7 Recruitment of follicles followed by selection of the dominant follicle and atresia of the remaining follicles.

continues developing. All others stop growing and begin to recede in size, a process called atresia (Figure 2.7). These atretic follicles degenerate and do not grow again. The single surviving follicle, also referred to as the dominant follicle, continues to develop. At a later stage of development a fluid filled cavity develops within the follicle and the oocyte becomes suspended in this cavity (Figure 2.8). The oocyte is still surrounded by cells which are now known as the cumulus oophorus. At this stage the follicle is known as the Graffian follicle. Following a hormonal stimulus from the pituitary gland (to be described in a later section) the follicle ruptures to release the oocyte together with its surrounding cumulus cells, and this process is known as ovulation (Figure 2.9).

The released oocyte enters the fallopian tube and fertilization normally takes place there. It is presently thought that the oocyte can only be fertilized within 12–24 hours of ovulation. Spermatozoa should already be there in the fallopian tubes at the time of ovulation or get there within 12–24 hours. The ruptured follicle collapses and is filled with blood. This follicle still continues to develop and forms another structure called the corpus luteum. The corpus luteum degenerates after about two weeks if the woman does not become pregnant in that cycle. If she becomes pregnant, the corpus luteum continues to produce hormones (primarily progesterone) which are important for the survival of the pregnancy, by maintaining the endometrium, for the first few weeks. When it degenerates eventually it is called the corpus albicans (Figure 2.9). An ovarian cycle lasts 28 days on the average. It starts at some point during the development of the cohort of primordial follicles. Ovulation occurs halfway through the cycle (Day 14). If the woman does not become pregnant in that cycle, the corpus luteum begins to degenerate 3–4 days before the end of the cycle.

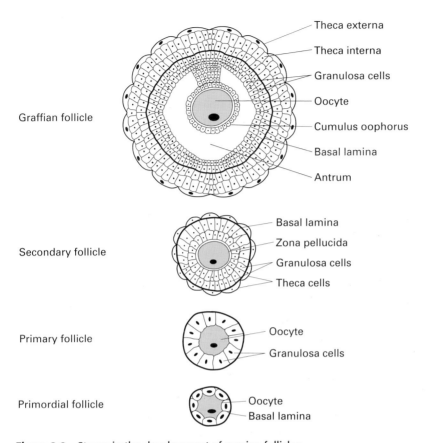

Figure 2.8   Stages in the development of ovarian follicles.

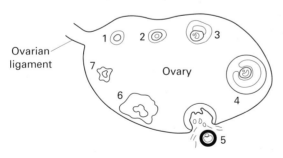

Figure 2.9   Section through an ovary showing follicular development until ovulation, corpus luteum formation and atresia: (1) primordial follicle; (2) primary follicle; (3) secondary follicle; (4) Graffian follicle; (5) ovulation of oocyte–cumulus complex; (6) corpus luteum; and (7) corpus albicantes.

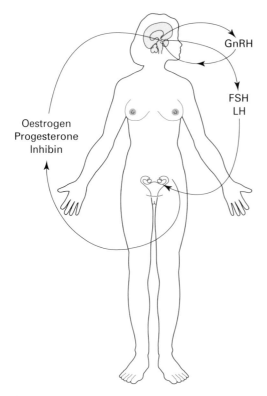

Figure 2.10 Endocrine control of reproductive function. The hypothalamus produces gonadotrophin releasing hormone (GnRH) which stimulates release of follicle stimulating hormone (FSH) and luteinizing hormone (LH) from the pituitary gland. FSH and LH then act on the ovary resulting in the production of oestrogen which exerts feedback control on hypothalamic and pituitary secretion of GnRH, FSH and LH respectively.

Hormonal control of the ovarian cycle

The hypothalamus and the pituitary gland are involved in the control of ovarian function just as in males (see Chapter 1). However, the feedback control mechanisms are more complex than those found in the male. Gonadotrophin releasing hormone (GnRH) is produced by the hypothalamus and stimulates the pituitary to release follicle stimulating hormone (FSH) and luteinizing hormone (LH) (Figure 2.10). FSH stimulates the growth and development of ovarian follicles. LH stimulates cells in these follicles to produce two other hormones. The first hormone is oestrogen and is produced right from the beginning of the ovarian cycle. The second hormone, progesterone, is produced by the corpus luteum after ovulation. LH also contributes to the development of the follicles. In the early part of the cycle oestrogen that is produced by the follicles acts on the hypothalamus and pituitary

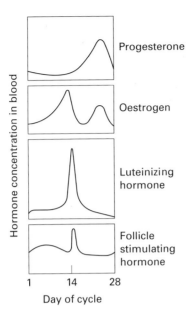

Figure 2.11 Hormonal interrelationships during the menstrual cycle.

to decrease their hormonal secretions (i.e. GnRH, FSH and LH). One consequence of this is that the developing follicles are starved of FSH. However, one follicle, the dominant follicle, is able to continue developing despite the lower FSH levels. This is because it has a higher density of FSH receptors and is able to make more efficient use of ambient FSH levels unlike the others. All other follicles in the cohort undergo atresia. Towards the middle of the cycle the increasing and sustained oestrogen levels have another type of effect on the pituitary. This time, instead of decreasing the secretion of FSH and LH, oestrogen stimulates the pituitary suddenly to produce large amounts of these hormones for a short while. This sudden surge in the production of FSH and LH by the pituitary is such that the concentrations of these hormones in the blood increase dramatically. The increase is more pronounced for LH. The LH surge induces final maturational changes in the oocyte. It also leads to weakening of the follicle wall and its eventual rupture about 36 hours later. The temporal relationship of these hormonal events to each other is depicted in Figure 2.11. Oestrogen and progesterone have their main effects on the endometrium as will be described shortly.

Menstrual cycle

The endometrium undergoes cyclical changes in concert with those of the ovarian cycle. Menstruation occurs at the beginning of the cycle and the first day of

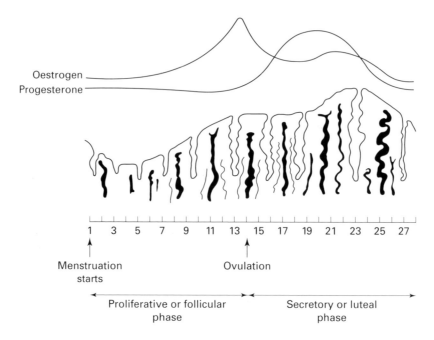

Figure 2.12 Correlation between oestrogen and progesterone concentrations during the menstrual cycle and endometrial development.

bleeding is regarded as Day 1 of the cycle. The superficial layers of the endometrium are shed in the following days and the total number of days of bleeding (two to seven days) varies from one individual to another. At the end of menstruation, only a thin layer of the endometrium remains but it starts to rebuild itself and increase in thickness soon afterwards (Figure 2.12). This increase in thickness is initially stimulated by oestrogen, which is produced in the ovary. Later, progesterone brings about further growth of the endometrium and changes that will favour establishment of pregnancy. If pregnancy does not occur, growth of the endometrium stops and it starts to break down. Onset of the menstrual period marks the end of the current cycle and the beginning of a new cycle.

The 'phases'

Certain terminology are used to describe different segments of the ovarian and menstrual cycles. The follicular phase describes the first half of the ovarian cycle. This is the time during which ovarian follicles develop. The luteal phase refers to the second half of the ovarian cycle. This marks the time during which the corpus luteum develops and functions. Ovulation demarcates the follicular from the luteal phases (Figure 2.13). The first half of the menstrual cycle is the proliferative phase.

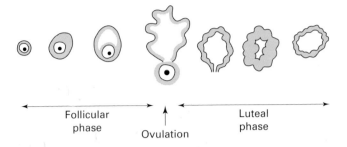

Follicular phase   Ovulation   Luteal phase

Figure 2.13 Ovulation as a marker of the transition from follicular to luteal development.

During this time the endometrium increases in size mainly as a result of an increase in the number of cells it contains (Figure 2.12). The proliferative phase of the menstrual cycle corresponds to the follicular phase of the ovarian cycle. Ovulation also signals the end of the proliferative phase. The latter half of the menstrual cycle is called the secretory phase. The endometrium increases in size during this time as a result of accumulation of fluid and secretion of mucin by glands. The secretory phase corresponds to the luteal phase of the ovarian cycle. The interrelationships of the ovarian and menstrual cycles and the relevant hormones are shown in Figure 2.12.

Cycle length and timing of events

For a woman who has a 28-day cycle, both ovarian and menstrual cycles start on Day 1. The LH/FSH surge takes place on Day 12 and ovulation occurs on Day 14. The proliferative (or follicular) phase lasts 14 days. The interval between ovulation and menstruation (luteal or secretory phase) is 14 days. It is important to note that menstruation commences 14 days after ovulation and this is constant irrespective of the overall length of the female's menstrual/ovarian cycle. This is illustrated in Figure 2.14. It is possible to estimate how long a female can remain fertile during each menstrual cycle. If sexual intercourse takes place during that 'fertile period' there is a high probability that both the oocyte and spermatozoa will be present in the tube at the same time. It however does not guarantee that the spermatozoa will fertilize the released oocyte. Since spermatozoa can survive in the female genital tract for about 72 hours it means that sexual intercourse during the three days before an expected ovulation and up to 24 hours (1 day) after the ovulation can result in pregnancy. The fertile period is therefore four days and extends from Day 11 to Day 15 in a 28-day cycle. Of course the nearer sexual intercourse is to the time of ovulation the greater the chance of viable spermatozoa being present in the tube at ovulation. It is also possible for fertilization to occur if intercourse takes place

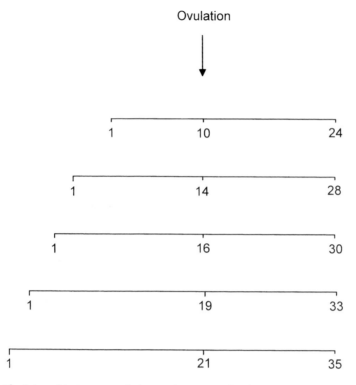

Figure 2.14 The interval between ovulation and menstruation is constant irrespective of the menstrual cycle length.

slightly outside this time frame. One reason for this may be that of the gametes (oocyte and spermatozoa) remaining viable for longer periods of time than presently documented. Another possibility is that the female ovulates earlier than usual. This is however no problem for couples who have been trying for pregnancy. Those who are trying to avoid pregnancy should use effective contraceptives for intercourse that takes place anytime from five days to the expected ovulation to two days afterwards.

Cervical mucus

The cervix is the major source of mucus that is found issuing from the external os at different times during the menstrual cycle. A small amount of secretion originates from sites higher up in the female genital canal such as the endometrium and fallopian tubes. Water constitutes 90% of the mucus followed by mucin, white blood cells and dead endometrial and cervical cells. The ovarian hormones influence the quality of this mucus. Oestrogen stimulates the cervix to produce a

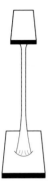

Figure 2.15 Pre-ovulatory cervical mucus can be made to stretch between two glass slides or two fingers.

copious watery mucus. The mucus is clear just like raw egg white, feels slippery and can stretch (Figure 2.15). This is usually found around the midcycle, a few days before ovulation and marks the height of the activity of oestrogen on the genital organs. About 5 ml of mucus a day is secreted at this time and this type of cervical mucus is said to be 'favourable'. The woman is usually able to notice this type of cervical mucus or can be taught to recognize its appearance. Some couples use the appearance of this mucus to time sexual intercourse for conception or contraception. Following ovulation the corpus luteum is formed and begins to secrete progesterone. This hormone inhibits production of the watery type of mucus. Instead, a thick whitish viscid secretion is produced by the cervix.

A number of functions have been ascribed to the cervix and its mucus such as control of the entry of spermatozoa into the uterine cavity. The viscid mucus that is found during the time of progesterone secretion does not allow spermatozoa to enter the cervical canal. Even when the mucus is favourable the cervix still exerts a selective function on entry of spermatozoa; only spermatozoa with normal shape and exhibiting rapid straight line movement succeed in gaining entrance into the canal. Once in the canal the cervical mucus protects spermatozoa from vaginal acidity and from being destroyed by white blood cells that normally engulf foreign material. The mucus nourishes the spermatozoa during the time they reside in the cervical canal. The mucus filled crypts act as storage for spermatozoa. Spermatozoa that swim into these crypts can be kept alive for up to three days. It is presently believed that spermatozoa leave these crypts at intervals and ascend the genital tract where they may encounter an ovulated oocyte and succeed in fertilizing it. Finally, cervical mucus initiates changes in the spermatozoa that prepare them for fertilization. This process is called capacitation. Cervical mucus can be evaluated and a number of tests are now available for checking the quality of the mucus and its interaction with spermatozoa. These will be discussed in later chapters.

Applied concepts

- When the Graffian follicle ruptures at the time of ovulation, some bleeding occurs from the follicle and the blood irritates the delicate lining membrane of the abdominal and pelvic cavities called the peritoneum thereby causing pain. This may be the cause of the so-called ovulation pain. It is a relatively reliable sign of the occurrence of ovulation but may not be felt by every female in every ovarian cycle.
- The menstrual cycle length varies from one individual to another. Furthermore, each female rarely has constant cycle lengths. Provided the menstrual cycle length falls within the range of 24–35 days there should be no need for anxiety. It is only when the interval is shorter than this or becomes much longer that the female should be evaluated especially if there is difficulty in achieving pregnancy.
- It was previously thought that each ovary took turns to ovulate each month but now it is known that the side of ovulation is random.

BIBLIOGRAPHY

Chard, T. & Grudzinskas, J. G. (Eds) (1994). *The Uterus.* Cambridge: Cambridge University Press.

Grudzinskas, J. G., Chapman, M. G., Chard, T. & Djahanbakhch, O. (1994). *The Fallopian Tube, Clinical and Surgical Aspects.* London: Springer-Verlag.

Grudzinskas, J. G. & Yovich, J. L. (Eds) (1995). *Gametes – The Oocyte.* Cambridge: Cambridge University Press.

Johnson, M. & Everitt, B. (2000). *Essential Reproduction,* 5th edn. London: Blackwell Science.

Knobil, E. & Neill, J. D. (Eds), Greenwald, G. S., Markert, C. L. & Pfaff, D. W. (Associate Eds) (1994). *The Physiology of Reproduction,* 2nd edn. New York: Raven Press.

Rowe, P. J., Comhaire, F. H., Hargreave, T. B. & Mellows, H. J. (1993). *WHO Manual for the Standardized Investigation and Diagnosis of the Infertile Couple.* Cambridge: Cambridge University Press.

World Health Organization (1992). *WHO Laboratory Manual for the Examination of Human Semen and Sperm-Cervical Mucus Interaction,* 3rd edn. Cambridge: Cambridge University Press.

World Health Organization (1999). *WHO Laboratory Manual for the Examination of Human Semen and Sperm-Cervical Mucus Interaction,* 4th edn. Cambridge: Cambridge University Press.

3

Fertilization, implantation and early development

Introduction

Fertilization of the oocyte is one of the key events of conception. However, for this to happen, the spermatozoa has to undergo a difficult journey up the female genital tract from the hazardous vaginal environment, through the screening mechanisms of the cervix and traverse the relatively long distance of the uterine cavity and fallopian tubal lumen. With successful union of the male and female gametes the resulting embryo travels in the opposite direction to that of the sperm to arrive at the uterine cavity at a time, which if optimal, allows it to implant successfully in the endometrium. A knowledge of these events is important for understanding the mechanisms of various aetiological factors in infertility and approaches to their management.

Transport of spermatozoa in the female

Semen is deposited in the vagina at the time of ejaculation. As was mentioned in Chapter 1, the semen clots immediately after ejaculation. The clot however starts liquefying within a few minutes and is usually complete within 30 minutes. As liquefaction begins, spermatozoa start entering the cervical canal through the external os. If sexual intercourse takes place during the mid-cycle just prior to ovulation, the cervical mucus will be favourable (see Chapter 2). The mucus allows the movement of spermatozoa through the cervical canal and into the uterine cavity. At the same time some spermatozoa leave the cervical canal and enter the cervical crypts where, theoretically, they can survive for up to three days in the presence of a favourable mucus. At intervals, spermatozoa emerge from these crypts and ascend the rest of the cervical canal to reach the uterine cavity.

Not all spermatozoa in the ejaculate succeed in entering the cervical canal. In fact only about 1% or less do so. The rest perish in the vagina after about one to two hours due to the vaginal acidity. Most of the semen will flow out of the vagina when a woman stands up after sexual intercourse. This does not affect fertility and a

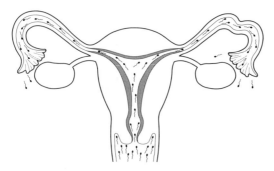

Figure 3.1   Sperm ingress into the female genital tract. It is not known for certain if there is a preferential entry of sperm into the fallopian tube that harbours the ovulated oocyte.

woman does not need to lie on the bed for long periods after intercourse. However, on empirical grounds a woman can lie flat on the bed for 30–60 minutes after intercourse before getting up, if the couple are anxious about their fertility and want to be sure they are not doing anything to jeopardise it. Having said this it must be emphasized that there is no scientific evidence to show that the woman's position during and after sexual intercourse affects her chances of conception. Couples are free to carry on as they wish. Spermatozoa reaching the uterine cavity swim upwards to enter both fallopian tubes (Figure 3.1). At present it is not known for certain if there is a stimulus (signal) that guides spermatozoa to the particular tube an ovulated oocyte will enter. If the spermatozoa happen to encounter an oocyte in the fallopian tube they will attempt to fertilize it.

The mature oocyte

The ovulated oocyte is still surrounded by the cumulus oophorus (see Chapter 2) (Figure 3.2). The oocyte itself has an outer shell called the zona pellucida and an inner membrane called the oolemma or vitelline membrane. The space between the zona pellucida and the oolemma is called the perivitelline space. The oolemma envelopes the cytoplasm of the oocyte (or ooplasm) which is a semi-fluid material. Various components of the cell are suspended in this ooplasm including the nucleus. It is the nucleus that contains a copy of the woman's genetic make-up. The polar body is found in the perivitelline space. This is a by-product of meiosis that begins in the oocyte while it is still developing inside the ovarian follicle. This type of cell division results in the reduction of the number of chromosomes in the oocyte by half. The other half of the chromosomes is contained in the first polar body. A similar chromosome reduction division occurs during the production of spermatozoa in the testis. At fertilization, the half (haploid) set of chromosomes in the sperm combines with that of the oocyte to restore the full (diploid) complement of

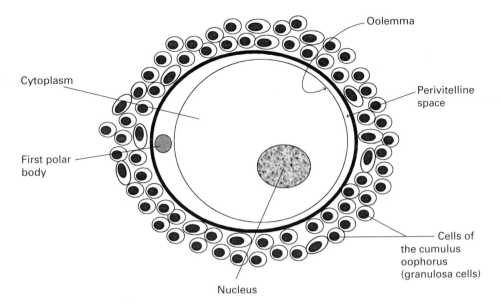

Figure 3.2   The oocyte-cumulus complex consisting of the oocyte and the surrounding granulosa cells, the latter of which form the cumulus oophorus.

chromosomes in the embryo. A second polar body is formed during fertilization and usually comes to lie beside the first polar body in the perivitelline space.

Fertilization

Before fertilization can occur, the cells of the cumulus oophorus have to be separated so that a pathway is created for spermatozoa to reach the oocyte. This process is carried out by the spermatozoa which release an enzyme, hyaluronidase, that breaks the connective tissue elements (bonds) holding the cells of the cumulus oophorus together. Several spermatozoa attach to the zona pellucida and attempt to pass through this layer and enter the perivitelline space. The first spermatozoon that succeeds in doing so and fusing with the oolemma fertilizes the oocyte. The oolemma then changes its nature so as to prevent any more spermatozoa from fusing with it and entering the ooplasm. Fertilization occurs within one hour or at most four hours of spermatozoa coming into contact with the oocyte. The first evidence of successful fertilization is the appearance of two pronuclei in the ooplasm about four to seven hours after fusion of the sperm with the oolemma (Figures 3.3 and 3.4). One pronucleus is formed by the nucleus of the oocyte while the other is formed by the nucleus of the spermatozoon. Later on, the fertilized oocyte divides into two cells and is now known as an embryo. Each cell then divides into two and so on. Not all the cells divide at the same rate. One of the cells in the two-cell

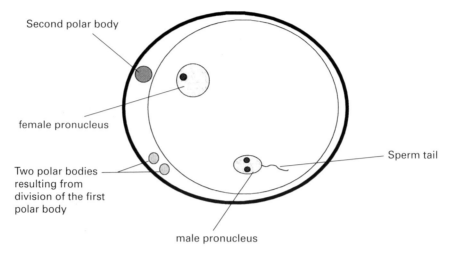

Figure 3.3 Diagram to show the two-pronuclear oocyte.

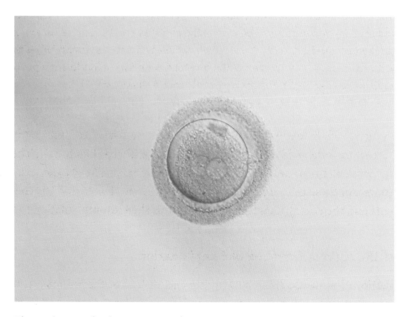

Figure 3.4 Photomicrograph of a two-pronuclear oocyte.

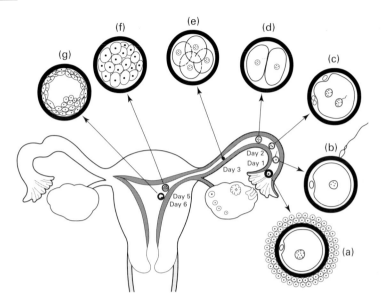

Figure 3.5 The upper female genital tract and ovaries showing key follicular developmental stages followed by ovulation, tubal pick-up of the ovulated oocyte, fertilization and early embryonic development: (a) the oocyte-cumulus complex is successfully picked up by the fallopian tube; (b) fertilization of the oocyte; (c) the two-pronuclear oocyte; (d) two cell embryo; (e) four cell embryo; (f) morulla; and (g) blastocyst.

embryo will divide first giving rise to an embryo with three cells followed by division of the other cell giving rise to a four-cell embryo (Figure 3.5). The division of the embryo continues. At some stage the embryo has 16 cells, then 32, then 64 and so on. All these cells are still contained within the shell formed by the zona pellucida and the embryo has to hatch out of this shell for implantation to take place.

Transport of the embryo, hatching and implantation

Fertilization takes place usually in the outer half of the fallopian tube called the ampulla. It however takes five days for the embryo to reach the uterine cavity (Figure 3.5). During transit through the fallopian tube, the embryo is nourished by secretions from the tube. There comes a stage during transit when the embryo has so many cells that it appears like a ball of cells. At this stage it is called a morula. Fluid then accumulates within this ball of cells and a fluid filled cavity, called the blastocoele, appears at the centre. The embryo is now called a blastocyst (Figure 3.5).

It is the blastocyst that implants in the endometrium. Prior to implantation the blastocyst hatches through the zona pellucida. This is achieved by the thinning of

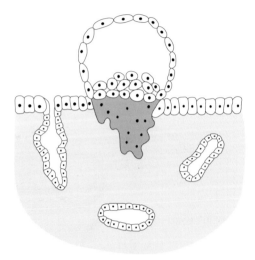

Figure 3.6   Section of the uterine wall showing the implanting embryo.

the zona pellucida by enzymes produced by the blastocyst. The blastocyst also contracts and expands until the zona pellucida cracks open and releases the embryo. The embryo then begins to signal its presence to the mother. It is important that the maternal system recognizes the presence of an embryo so as to avoid setting off processes that lead to menstruation. The embryo signals to the mother using various chemical and physical stimuli. The most well known chemical signal is the secretion of human chorionic gonadotrophin (hCG). hCG is absorbed into the mother's blood system to reach the ovaries where it prevents the corpus luteum from regressing. It also stimulates the corpus luteum to increase production of progesterone and oestrogen because it is these hormones that maintain the uterine endometrium and increase its size. Progesterone and oestrogen also have several other positive effects on the establishment of pregnancy.

The embryo implants in the endometrium, seven days after ovulation, by sinking into a cleft in that layer (Figure 3.6). The endometrium then covers the embryo completely. The embryo soon establishes contact with the mother's blood stream from which it extracts oxygen and nutrients through the placenta. The embryo also discharges its waste products into the mother's blood for removal through her urine. Subsequent growth and development of the conceptus is nothing short of miraculous; the embryo changes from a ball of cells into a human being with billions of cells and complex organ systems, all within a space of roughly nine months (Figure 3.7). The fetus and the placenta should have fully taken over production of progesterone and oestrogen from the corpus luteum before the end of the eighth week of pregnancy.

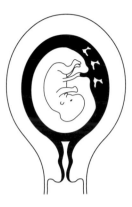

Figure 3.7   The fetus in late first trimester of pregnancy.

BIBLIOGRAPHY

Johnson, M. & Everitt, B. (2000). *Essential Reproduction*, 5th edn. London: Blackwell Science.

Knobil, E. & Neill, J. D. (Eds), Greenwald, G. S., Markert, C. L. & Pfaff, D. W. (Associate Eds) (1994). *The Physiology of Reproduction*, 2nd edn. New York: Raven Press.

4

Male factor problems

Introduction

The contribution of the male partner to infertility in the couple will be considered in this chapter using the system of classification proposed by the World Health Organization (Table 4.1) (Rowe et al., 1993). The characteristics of a normal semen sample were introduced in Chapter 1. Further details will be provided when discussing the evaluation of infertile couples in Chapter 6. Male factor problems commonly manifest through an alteration of one or more semen parameters and the following terminology are used to describe the changes.

- *Azoospermia* – spermatozoa cannot be found in a semen sample.
- *Aspermia* – no semen sample was ejaculated at orgasm.
- *Necrozoospermia* – all spermatozoa in the semen sample are dead.
- *Globozoospermia* – none of the spermatozoa have an acrosomal cap.
- *Oligozoospermia* – the concentration of spermatozoa is less than 20 million/ml of the ejaculate.
- *Asthenozoospermia* – less than 50% of spermatozoa in the semen sample exhibit forward motility.
- *Teratozoospermia* – the proportion of spermatozoa with normal shape is less than 30%.

A semen sample may at times have more than one of the last three abnormal profiles necessitating a combination of terminology. Thus oligoasthenoteratozoospermia describes a semen sample with all three abnormalities. Likewise, the presence of two abnormalities will require the use of the appropriate terminology, for example, asthenoteratozoospermia.

Sexual and/or ejaculatory dysfunction

Infrequent sexual intercourse

Some couples may present with infertility because they do not have intercourse frequently enough to ensure that spermatozoa are present in the female genital tract

Table 4.1. Male diagnostic categories

Sexual and/or ejaculatory dysfunction	Male accessory gland infection
Immunological cause	Endocrine cause
No demonstrable abnormality	Idiopathic oligozoospermia
Isolated seminal plasma abnormalities	Idiopathic asthenozoospermia
Iatrogenic cause	Idiopathic teratozoospermia
Systemic cause	Obstructive azoospermia
Congenital abnormalities	Idiopathic cryptozoospermia
Acquired testicular damage	Idiopathic azoospermia
Varicocoele	

Source: From Rowe et al. (1993, 2000).

around the time of ovulation. The optimal frequency of sexual intercourse is unknown. However, if it happens at least three times a week there is a reasonable chance that this will be adequate for conception. Patterns of sexual activity amongst couples show a wide variation. Some may not maintain a high frequency of sexual intercourse for a long period of time for many reasons. It is important for these particular couples to ensure that they increase their sexual activity around the time of ovulation.

Wrong timing of sexual intercourse

Some couples may concentrate their sexual activity at the wrong time of the menstrual/ovarian cycle. It has been known for a couple to have sexual intercourse only at the time of menstruation or soon afterwards because they believed that that was when the woman was most fertile.

Impotence or ejaculatory failure

Impotence, or erectile dysfunction, is an inability to have or maintain an erection long enough to allow sexual intercourse to take place. In ejaculatory failure, the man may have an erection but is unable to ejaculate during sexual intercourse. Both may be caused by psychological factors, but these are not well understood at present. The problems can also be caused by chronic diseases such as diabetes mellitus, multiple sclerosis, thyroid disorders, epilepsy, atherosclerosis and renal failure. Spinal cord injury is also a well-known cause. Certain major abdominal and pelvic operations for cancer can damage nerves supplying the male genital organs and cause problems with erection or ejaculation. There is also a long list of drugs that may be implicated (Table 4.2).

Table 4.2. Drugs involved in the causation of impotence and ejaculatory dysfunction

Sedatives and antidepressants	
Amitriptyline	Monoamine oxidase inhibitors
Chlordiazepoxide	Perphenazine
Chlorpromazine	Phenelzine sulphate
Diazepam	Thioridazine
Imipramine	Trifluoperazine hydrochloride
Antihypertensive agents	
Clonidine	Prazosin hydrochloride
Guanethidine sulphate	Propranolol
Hydralazine	Reserpine
Methyldopa	Spironolactone
Metoprolol	Thiazide diuretics
Phenoxybenzamine hydrochloride	
Drugs of abuse	
Alcohol	Nicotine
Cocaine	Methadone
Codeine	Meperidine
Heroin	
Others	
Clofibrate	Digoxin
Cimetidine	Ketoconazole

Source: Adapted from Meniru & Akagbosu (1997).

Premature ejaculation

Ejaculation is said to be premature if it takes place within a short time of sexual arousal. It can only be regarded as a cause of infertility if ejaculation occurs outside the vagina. If intravaginal ejaculation always takes place, other causes for the infertility have to be looked for. At the same time the couple in question can seek psychosexual assistance to enable the man to achieve better control over the timing of his ejaculation so as to allow his wife adequate time to enjoy the sexual act and hopefully reach an orgasm.

Retrograde ejaculation

As was described in Chapter 1, the bladder sphincters are closed at the time of ejaculation thereby preventing semen from passing backwards into the bladder. Diseases such as diabetes mellitus and multiple sclerosis may impair the closure of these sphincters leading to retrograde ejaculation. Operations around the bladder neck such as prostatectomy (removal of part of or the whole prostate gland) can also cause this problem. Some of the drugs listed in Table 4.2 have been implicated on occasions. Since semen is propelled backwards into the bladder, rather than forwards and out of the penis, there is no intravaginal deposition of semen.

Extravaginal ejaculation

Deposition of semen outside the vagina can occur not only in cases of premature ejaculation but also in men who have severe hypospadias or epispadias. In these latter conditions the opening of the urethra is not at the tip of the penis but somewhere along the shaft of the penis due to failed development of the rest of the urethra. If the opening is high up on the shaft (i.e. at the root of the penis) semen will be ejaculated outside the vagina. These are rare causes of infertility nowadays because they are detectable at birth and can be corrected by surgery during childhood.

Immunological cause

The body normally produces antibodies to protect itself from foreign organisms such as bacteria and viruses. Occasionally antibodies against spermatozoa may be produced by the body and they will be found in semen and/or blood. These antisperm antibodies can be produced when there is damage to the testes, infection of the testes and surrounding tissues or obstruction to the transport of spermatozoa along the male genital tract. Antisperm antibodies may bind to spermatozoa and prevent them from moving. The antibodies can also bind several spermatozoa together to form a clump. Even if the motility of spermatozoa is not impaired, these antisperm antibodies may prevent the fertilization of the egg by affected spermatozoa that reach the fallopian tubes. However, the presence of antisperm antibodies does not always signify infertility because many men with these antibodies are able to impregnate their wives. In other words antisperm antibodies reduce fertility but do not prevent conception in every case where they are found; they are a relative rather than an absolute cause of infertility.

No demonstrable abnormality

There are many men in whom no cause is found for the infertile state existing in the couple. Their semen parameters appear normal. In-depth questioning does not uncover any problems with sexual intercourse and its timing or other causes of infertility. Examination of the man also fails to show up any problem. If the woman likewise does not have any obvious problem the couple are said to have unexplained infertility.

Isolated seminal plasma abnormalities

In some men, the spermatozoa appear normal in all aspects but they might adhere together as if there were antisperm antibodies in the semen. However, tests will fail to show any of the known classes of antisperm antibodies. Some other men may have low volume ejaculates, acidic or very alkaline semen or more white blood cells than normal. All these men are said to have isolated seminal plasma abnormalities. Attempts are always made to find out the cause of these problems such as accessory gland dysfunction and infection.

Iatrogenic cause

Production of spermatozoa in the testes may be depressed by drugs used for the treatment of certain ailments. Such drugs include hormones, sulphasalazine, cimetidine, nitrofurantoin, niridazole, spironolactone and colchicine (Rowe et al., 1993, 2000). Anticancer (cytotoxic) drugs are strong depressants of testicular function and production of spermatozoa may never return to normal levels following completion of treatment with some of the drugs, for example alkylating agents (cyclophosphamide, busulphan, chlorambucil, etc.). There are many other drugs that have similar depressant effects. Infertility could be a result of complications from certain operations, such as prostatectomy, and from childhood operations on the male genital tract. Repair of inguinal hernias or hydrocoeles, and other genital or inguinal operations may damage the vasa deferentia leading to their partial or complete blockage and possibly antisperm antibody formation. Vasectomy is another such operation, but it should be noted that this operation is designed for permanent contraception. However, some men may, sometime afterwards, wish to have the operation reversed to allow them to have more children. Also, anabolic steroids used by some athletes to boost their performance can have the significant undesirable side-effect of depression of fertility.

Systemic cause

Diabetes and other diseases that affect the function of nerves in the body may cause impotence, retrograde ejaculation or no ejaculation at all. Tuberculosis may lead to infection of the epididymides and prostate gland. Any illness that causes high fever can depress production of spermatozoa for up to six months. General anaesthesia, major surgery, burns and head injury can also cause decreased sperm production. Alcohol and other drugs of abuse adversely affect production of spermatozoa. The same goes for toxins that may be found in some environments and occupations such as lead, cadmium, mercury, pesticides and herbicides. There is presently no agreement on whether or not tobacco smoking depresses production of spermatozoa but marijuana does depress fertility.

Congenital abnormalities

Most male infants are born with both testes already in the scrotum. Occasionally some may be born with one or both testes still within the abdomen or somewhere along the line of descent to the scrotum. This is more common in premature infants. Although descent may continue after birth and both testes enter the scrotum soon after delivery, it is always important that the baby is seen by a paediatrician who will ensure that the most appropriate treatment is given. Treatment may be by the administration of drugs or through surgery. Testes that have not descended into the scrotum by adolescence may not produce spermatozoa at all or produce very deficient amounts. Optimal production of spermatozoa takes place when the testes are slightly cooler than the rest of the body and this is achieved when they are within the scrotum. Undescended testes can become traumatized if lying in the groin and testicular cancer is much more common in men with undescended testes than others.

The vasa deferentia and/or seminal vesicles fail to develop in some individuals especially those who have or are carriers of cystic fibrosis. Such individuals have azoospermia because spermatozoa that are produced in the testes cannot be transported to the ejaculatory duct and urethra. Some chromosomal abnormalities may lead to non-functioning testes. Other genetic abnormalities could be associated with functioning testes but the quality of the spermatozoa is poor. Some of these genetic abnormalities can be transmitted to the male offspring of men with such abnormalities.

Acquired testicular damage

The virus that causes mumps can also infect the testes in 20–30% of males who contract this infection after puberty. There is a high likelihood of testicular damage in such circumstances and this may be irreversible in some cases. Other infections that have been associated with male infertility (Rowe et al. 2000) include tuberculosis, bilharziasis, gonorrhoea, chlamydia, filariasis, typhoid, influenza, brucellosis and syphilis. Injury to the testes from accidents or even operations can also depress the production of spermatozoa. In torsion of the testis, the testis twists on its cord thereby shutting off its blood supply. If this is diagnosed and untwisted by surgery within a short while the function of the testis may not be adversely affected.

Varicocoele

This is a condition in which the veins that drain the testes become dilated and engorged with blood due to a poor flow of blood away from the testes. The veins are said to be varicose (just like varicose veins of the legs). Varicocoeles are more common on the left side and are of different grades. Some may not be obvious and are only detected using specialized equipment such as ultrasound. Others may be so large that they can be felt through the scrotum. In fact some people have described large varicocoeles in the scrotum as feeling like a bag of worms. Although there is still some controversy, many authorities in fertility management believe that varicocoeles depress the production of spermatozoa by the testes but there are also many men with varicocoeles who have normal semen parameters on analysis. About 18% of male partners in infertile couples have varicocoeles and poor semen parameters are found in two-thirds of them. Varicocoeles are believed to increase the scrotal temperature. Furthermore, the poor drainage of blood away from the testes may impair the function of the testes.

Male accessory gland infection

The accessory glands (seminal vesicles, prostate and Cowper's glands) may become infected with organisms that cause the sexually transmitted diseases such as gonorrhoea, syphilis, chlamydia and non-specific urethritis. Urinary tract infections can secondarily affect the accessory glands. These infections may affect the contribution of these glands to seminal fluid. They can also extend to the vas deferens and epididymis, and cause their blockage. Testicular infection will affect the production of spermatozoa as well as lead to the production of antisperm antibodies.

Endocrine cause

Lack of gonadotrophin stimulation of the testes may be the cause of infertility in some men. This can be caused by a broad range of disorders that prevent the secretion of FSH and LH by the pituitary. At times the problem may be higher up, affecting the secretion of gonadotrophin releasing hormone by the hypothalamus. The disorders are either congenital or acquired. The first task is to identify the primary cause and treat if possible. Another endocrine problem that may be associated with male factor infertility is excessive secretion of another pituitary hormone called prolactin. At times it may be that there is a tumour in the pituitary that is causing the uncontrolled secretion of this hormone.

Unexplained poor semen parameters

In about 25% of male partners in infertile couples there is no cause found to explain the poor semen parameters. The word idiopathic is used to indicate this unexplained nature of the finding as follows:

- *Idiopathic oligozoospermia* – unexplained low concentration of spermatozoa (less than 20 million/ml).
- *Idiopathic asthenozoospermia* – unexplained low motility (less than 25% of spermatozoa are showing rapid straight line motion).
- *Idiopathic teratozoospermia* – unexplained low concentration of normal looking spermatozoa.
- *Idiopathic cryptozoospermia* – unexplained absence of spermatozoa from the semen sample during routine semen analysis. However, after centrifugation of the semen sample a few spermatozoa are seen.
- *Idiopathic azoospermia* – unexplained total absence of spermatozoa from the ejaculate.

Obstructive azoospermia

Obstruction to the flow of spermatozoa from the testis to the exterior results in azoospermia. Such obstruction can be caused by blockage of the epididymis or congenital absence of both vasa deferentia. Other causes include blockage of the ejaculatory duct and vasectomy. Inflammatory response to infection of the male genital tract may lead to tissue damage that is severe enough to block the tract.

Conclusion

The relative importance of causes of male factor infertility varies from country to country and also within countries. Table 4.3 shows the distribution of these diagnostic categories in a population of infertile couples. In nearly half of the men no obvious cause for the infertility was found and their semen parameters were normal. About one-quarter of patients had poor semen parameters but no cause was found (i.e. idiopathic abnormal semen). Varicocoele had the next largest representation (12.3% of patients) and the semen parameters were poor in all patients in that group. Patients with endocrine and other causes were relatively few in number.

Table 4.3. Distribution of male factor problems in a group of 7057 infertile couples

Male factor problem	Percentage
No demonstrable cause (normal semen and sexual/ejaculatory function)	48.5
Idiopathic abnormal semen (no cause for abnormal semen parameters)	26.4
Varicocoele	12.3
Infectious factors	6.6
Immunological factors	3.1
Other acquired factors	2.6
Congenital factors	2.1
Sexual factors	1.7
Endocrine disturbances	0.6

Source: Adapted from Farley & Belsey (1988).

BIBLIOGRAPHY

Centola, G. M. & Ginsburg, K. A. (Eds) (1996). *Evaluation and Treatment of the Infertile Male.* Cambridge: Cambridge University Press.

Farley, T. M. M. & Belsey, F. H. (1988). The prevalence and aetiology of infertility. In *Biological Components of Fertility. Proceedings of the African Population Conference, Dakar, Senegal, November 1988.* International Union for the Scientific Study of Population, Liege, Belgium, vol. 1, pp. 2.1.15–2.1.30.

Forman, R., Gilmour-White, S. & Forman, N. (1996). *Drug Induced Infertility and Sexual Dysfunction.* Cambridge: Cambridge University Press.

Insler, V. & Lunenfeld, B. (Eds) (1993). *Infertility: Male and Female*, 2nd edn. Edinburgh: Churchill Livingstone.

McConnell, J. D. (1998). Diagnosis and treatment of male infertility. In *Textbook of Reproductive Medicine*, ed. B. R. Carr & R. E. Blackwell, 2nd edn, pp. 549–64. Stamford: Appleton & Lange.

Meniru, G. I. & Akagbosu, F. T. (1997). Patient selection and management. In *A Handbook of Intrauterine Insemination*, ed. G. I. Meniru, P. R. Brinsden & I. L. Craft, pp. 23–45. Cambridge: Cambridge University Press.

Rowe, P. J., Comhaire, F. H., Hargreave, T. B. & Mellows, H. J. (1993). *WHO Manual for the Standardized Investigation and Diagnosis of the Infertile Couple.* Cambridge: Cambridge University Press.

Rowe, P. J., Comhaire, F. H., Hargreave, T. B. & Mahmoud, A. M. A. (2000). *WHO Manual for the Standardized Investigation, Diagnosis and Management of the Infertile Male.* Cambridge: Cambridge University Press.

Speroff, L., Glass, R. H. & Kase, N. G. (1999). Male infertility. In *Clinical Gynecologic Endocrinology and Infertility*, 6th edn, pp. 1075–96. Baltimore: Lippincott Williams & Wilkins.

Tan, S. L. & Jacobs, H. S. (1991). *Infertility: Your Questions Answered.* Singapore: McGraw-Hill Book Company.

5

Female factor problems

Introduction

Female factor problems are said to be present, either alone or in combination with male factor problems, in about 50% of infertile couples. These female factor problems arise following disturbance of function of the female genital organs. Thus a problem related to the vagina may prevent or limit sexual intercourse. Likewise, the cervix may not allow spermatozoa to reach the upper genital tract. There may be problems with ovulation or tubal pick-up of the ovulated oocyte. These and other female factor problems will be considered in this chapter. The incidence of each problem varies from place to place and even amongst different social classes in an area. This is because certain problems are related to the individual's environment and lifestyle factors. Thus the pattern of sexual activity will influence the incidence of pelvic infection and resulting damage to the tubes. Some ovulatory problems are associated with either overeating and obesity or starvation and underweight. It is therefore not possible to give an incidence of these problems that will hold true in all parts of the world. The example in Figure 5.1, however, gives an idea of the relative importance of the various female factor problems to be described below.

The vagina

The role of the vagina in infertility is poorly understood. There do not appear to be many vaginal conditions that can cause infertility per se unless they prevent or limit sexual intercourse. An uncommon problem is vaginismus which is the condition in which there is involuntary contraction of the vaginal muscles to prevent insertion of the penis into the vagina. There is usually a psychological cause for vaginismus and the patient should be evaluated by a psychologist or counsellor. In a few instances there is a lesion in the pelvis which makes intercourse painful; the woman responds with vaginismus following initial painful episodes. There will be a need, at some stage during the treatment of vaginismus, for the patient to insert special plastic dilators into the vagina which will help her learn how to relax the vaginal

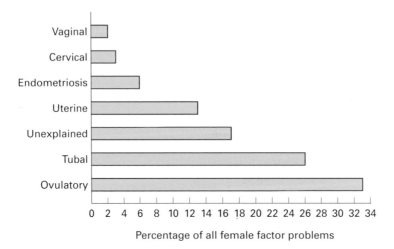

Figure 5.1   An estimate of the relative representation of the various female factor problems.

walls so that she can eventually allow insertion of the penis and hopefully have normal sexual intercourse. Any painful lesions of the vagina or pelvic organs, such as infection and endometriosis, will also limit the patient's sexual activity. Rarely, there may be a tough hymen that resists penetration of the vagina with the penis and has to be incised in the operating theatre. There have been occasional reports of couples living together for years without having vaginal intercourse because of such a rigid hymen and being too inexperienced to realize there was a problem and/or that a solution existed.

The cervix

Important functions of the cervix are described in Chapter 2. The cervix aids fertility by producing mucus that makes it possible for spermatozoa to move up the cervical canal. The mucus also nourishes spermatozoa that lodge in the crypts of the cervix. The cervix can cause or contribute to infertility in a number of ways. The quality of mucus that is produced at midcycle, just prior to ovulation, can be poor. For example, instead of being thin, watery, clear and stretchable it can be thick and form a plug at the external os preventing entry of spermatozoa into the cervical canal. In some patients, there may be little or no mucus production because a previous operation on the cervix, such as cone biopsy, destroyed or removed most of the mucus producing glands lining the cervical canal. There are times when the cervical mucus appears normal at midcycle but on analysis is found to contain antisperm antibodies. These antibodies can be produced by women, just

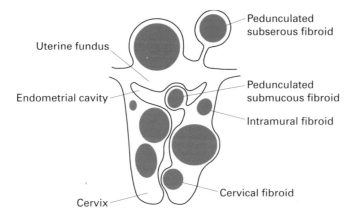

Figure 5.2   Uterine fibroids and distortion of the uterine cavity.

like men, and appear in the cervical mucus and/or blood. Long-standing infection of the cervical glands may lead to the presence of a large number of white blood cells in the mucus. These may engulf spermatozoa or produce chemical compounds that are toxic to them. Cervical mucus is said to be hostile if it is acidic, thicker in consistency than normal, contains more cells than usual or contains anti-sperm antibodies.

The uterus

Uterine factors may be the cause of infertility in a small proportion of patients.

Fibroids

Uterine fibroids are smooth muscle tumours of the uterus which are quite common, being found in up to 20% or more of females. The incidence is even higher in women of African descent. A more scientific term for fibroid is leiomyoma. Fibroids usually do not present symptoms and are discovered accidentally during routine pelvic examination for other reasons such as contraceptive advice or taking cervical smears. The association of fibroids with infertility is unclear and controversial. In rare instances there may be fibroids blocking the point of entry of both fallopian tubes into the uterine cavity. There may be just one fibroid in the uterus or several. The sizes also vary. When the uterus is riddled with several or large fibroids, the uterine cavity is likely to become distorted and hostile conditions exist such that conception becomes difficult (Figure 5.2). The presence of many fibroids bulging into the uterine cavity makes the endometrium unfavourable for implantation and the establishment of pregnancy. Having said this, it must be emphasized that there is no evidence that fibroids themselves cause infertility and millions of women conceive naturally and have normal pregnancies despite having one or more fibroids in their uterus. Blaming every fibroid uterus for the state of infertility is not helpful to patients especially as removal of the fibroids at operation does not necessarily mean a restoration of the woman's fertility. The infertile couple have to be investigated carefully to find out if more plausible causes for their infertility can be found.

Endometritis

Endometritis is an inflammation of the endometrium and may result from an infection with organisms such as the tuberculosis bacteria. Infertility can arise through the effects of toxins produced by the bacteria and abnormal secretions from the infected endometrial glands.

Asherman's syndrome

This is a condition in which parts of the uterine walls adhere together. In severe cases the uterine walls adhere fully together thereby obliterating the uterine cavity. Asherman's syndrome is caused by damage to the uterine walls soon after a pregnancy. One way this can happen is through excessive curettage (scraping) of the uterine wall during operations to remove pieces of retained placental tissue after delivery. The same complication can occur following termination of pregnancy or evacuation of retained products of conception after miscarriage. Implantation of the embryo is prevented in these patients because there is little or no endometrium left. Patients with Asherman's syndrome have either very scanty menstrual loss or none at all, in severe cases.

Uterine malformations

About 2–3% of females are born with a malformed uterus. Some of the malformations do not have any impact on the fertility of the woman while others do. These women may have problems with their menstrual periods such as scanty, heavy or irregular menstrual loss, or there may not be a communication between the uterine cavity and vagina to allow menstrual loss to drain out. Those women who become pregnant may have problems such as repeated midtrimester miscarriage (halfway through pregnancy) or repeated premature delivery. The baby may not lie in the normal position because of the abnormal shape of the mother's uterus. Some other babies are growth retarded. Uterine malformations, which can be detected with ultrasound scanning, can co-exist with malformations of the urinary tract. It is therefore important to investigate the urinary system carefully in all females found to have these uterine malformations. Common malformations of the uterus are shown in Figure 5.3

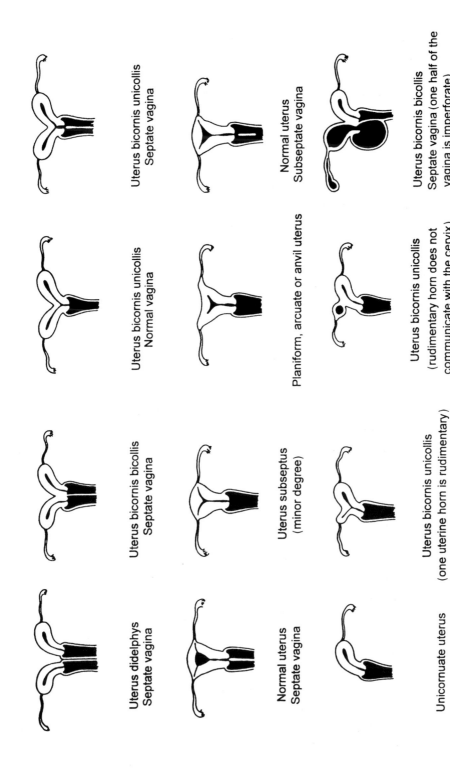

Figure 5.3 Congenital uterine anomalies. Adapted from Tindall (1987)

Uterus didelphys
Septate vagina

Uterus bicornis bicollis
Septate vagina

Uterus bicornis unicollis
Normal vagina

Uterus bicornis unicollis
Septate vagina

Normal uterus
Septate vagina

Uterus subseptus
(minor degree)

Planiform, arcuate or anvil uterus

Normal uterus
Subseptate vagina

Unicornuate uterus

Uterus bicornis unicollis
(one uterine horn is rudimentary)

Uterus bicornis unicollis
(rudimentary horn does not
communicate with the cervix)

Uterus bicornis bicollis
Septate vagina (one half of the
vagina is imperforate)

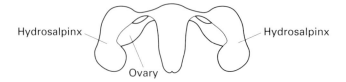

Figure 5.4   Bilateral hydrosalpinges.

The fallopian tubes

The fallopian tubes serve a vital role in procreation by providing the site for fertilization. Spermatozoa ascending the female genital tract enter the tubes from the uterine end while ovulated oocytes enter from the other end (i.e. the fimbrial end). Fertility problems arise if any factor interferes with this function. Infection in the lower genital tract (vagina and cervix) can spread to the tubes. Infection from any point in the lower abdomen and pelvis, especially the appendix during an attack of appendicitis, can also cause fertility problems. Gonorrhoea, chlamydia and pelvic tuberculosis are well known pelvic infections. Several other organisms have been implicated. Another name for infection in the pelvis is pelvic inflammatory disease or PID. The incidence of PID varies from community to community and reflects the pattern of sexual behaviour in an area. Where there is a high incidence of sexual activity, as for example in urban areas, the incidence of PID is also high. Promiscuity leads to rapid dissemination of infection within a geographical area and even outside it. Women who use the intrauterine contraceptive device (also known as the loop or coil) have a greater chance of having PID than others who do not use it. Infection after delivery, miscarriage or termination of pregnancy can also affect the tubes.

Tubal blockage can arise following an attack of PID especially if the infection is not treated promptly or eradicated completely. The risk of tubal blockage increases with the number of such attacks. If the blockage is at the fimbrial end of the tube, secretions may accumulate within the tube causing the obstructed end of the tube to balloon out and form what is known as a hydrosalpinx (Figure 5.4). Even if the tubes are not blocked their function may become compromised because cells that line the inside of the tubes can be damaged during the infection. Furthermore, adhesions (scar tissue) tend to form outside the fallopian tubes and restrict their movement. Adhesions can also pull away the tubes from their normal position.

A damaged tube that is not completely blocked may allow fertilization to take place within it but prevents the timely movement of the embryo down the tube and into the uterine cavity. This may lead to implantation occurring in the tube rather than in the uterine cavity thereby leading to ectopic pregnancy. Treatment of tubal ectopic pregnancies used to be mainly by removal of the affected tube(s). If both tubes were removed or one was removed but the remaining one was already badly damaged, infertility will result.

The function of the fallopian tubes can also be compromised following pelvic or abdominal operations. These operations can lead to the formation of adhesions in the pelvis. The adhesions cause infertility by constricting (thereby closing) the tubes or drawing them away from their normal position in the pelvis, the latter preventing normal oocyte pick up mechanisms of the tubes from functioning effectively. The fimbrial end of the tube can be buried in adhesions effectively blocking the tube. Infertile women are prone to having unnecessary operations performed on them. The unfortunate consequence of adhesion formation in the pelvis after such operations make these women even less likely to conceive naturally. The fact that has to be borne in mind by both patients and their doctors is that the pelvis does not readily forgive any intrusion, be it surgical or otherwise. It responds promptly by forming adhesions on and around pelvic organs whose integrity was breached. The mere touching of the pelvic organs with gloved hands or the wrong instruments can cause adhesion formation. Exposure of the organs to dry air during these operations will also damage their natural coverings. It is impossible to completely prevent bleeding during or after operations and any blood that is left behind in the pelvis can lead to the formation of adhesions. Once these adhesions form they are difficult to eradicate completely since they reform after operation; re-operation can even worsen the situation.

Patients must be made aware of this fact; such knowledge allows them to demand the highest quality of care in the management of their infertile condition. Any proposed operation involving the pelvic organs, especially in infertile women, must be discussed fully with the woman. The benefits of such surgery must have been documented in the scientific literature and the patient is right to demand to be shown such published reports. Furthermore, the benefit of the proposed operation should outweigh any risk of adhesion formation. Only clinicians who have special or sub-speciality training and experience in infertility surgery should be performing these operations.

The ovaries

Failure of ovulation (called anovulation) is found in more than a quarter of women in infertile relationships. There are many causes of anovulation and some are treatable while others are not. The main causes are summarized in Table 5.1. A more extensive list can be found in suitable texts.

Hypogonadotrophic hypogonadism

Just like in the male, there is a group of disorders that result in a lack of or deficient production of either gonadotrophin releasing hormone (GnRH) or follicle

Table 5.1. The main causes of anovulation

Hypogonadotrophic hypogonadism
Ovarian failure
Polycystic ovary syndrome
Weight loss/strenuous exercise
Hyperprolactinaemia

---

stimulating hormone (FSH) and luteinizing hormone (LH). Since there is no stimulation of their ovaries by FSH and LH, such women do not produce mature follicles or ovulate and their plasma oestrogen concentration is very low. The endometrium also does not go through the usual monthly cyclical developmental changes.

Ovarian failure

As was stated in Chapter 2, the female is born with all the oocytes she will ever ovulate already present in her ovaries. However, the number of oocytes begins to decrease, without being ovulated, from her fifth month in the womb, through the process known as atresia. By the time she is 25 years of age she only has about 60 000 oocytes remaining in her ovaries. By 40 years 8000 oocytes remain. As more oocytes degenerate in the ovary and the woman becomes older her fertility drops. This is because the oocytes remaining in the ovaries at that time are older and do not respond well to FSH and LH. In an attempt to improve this poor ovarian response the pituitary produces more FSH and LH but this does not have the desired effect and fewer oocytes continue to be ovulated. There comes a time when ovarian response is so poor that no more oocytes are ovulated. Normally this should occur when the woman is about 50 years old. The menstrual periods stop and the woman is said to be menopausal. Ovarian failure is normal in this context because it occurs at the expected age.

There are some females whose ovaries fail at an earlier age. If this happens before the age of 40 years they are said to have premature ovarian failure or premature menopause. This problem affects 1–5% of females in the general population and is caused by infections such as mumps, previous operations around the ovaries such as hysterectomy and some drugs used for treating cancers (cytotoxic drugs). The ovaries can also fail if they are irradiated during radiotherapy of cancers that affect organs that are close to the ovaries. The ovaries of individuals with certain chromosomal abnormalities, for example Turner's syndrome, may not contain many oocytes and fail even before the female has her first menstrual period. The most common causes of premature ovarian failure are the autoimmune disorders that may be found in up to 30% of patients. The woman produces antibodies against certain cells in her body, which may include the ovarian cells. In simple terms the woman's immune system does not recognize the cells of the ovaries as belonging to her and so attacks them just as it would attack any foreign body such as bacteria and viruses. A last group of patients do not have any obvious cause for their ovarian failure.

An early stage in the development of ovarian failure could be what is currently called resistant ovary syndrome. Here, the FSH and LH concentrations in blood begin to increase as the woman stops ovulating. However, at sporadic intervals she may ovulate spontaneously and anecdotal reports of pregnancy occurring in such circumstances have been made in the scientific literature. Much remains unknown about this syndrome including the fact that it may have an aetiology distinct from that of ovarian failure.

Females with ovarian failure are incapable of having children using their oocytes but they can still have children using oocytes that are donated by others with normal ovarian function.

Polycystic ovary syndrome

This is a condition in which there are several tiny cysts in the ovaries (Figure 5.5) coupled with the presence of one or more complaints such as complete cessation of the menstrual periods, irregular and/or long intervals between periods, obesity, excessive growth of body hair, greasy skin and acne. The ovaries tend to be larger than normal. These so-called cysts are not the sort of cysts that grow as ovarian tumours. Rather, they represent ovarian follicles that fail to complete their development apparently due to relatively low levels of FSH. The cause of this syndrome is unknown but it may be genetic. There seems to be a derangement in the hormonal activities of the ovaries and some other glands in the body. For example, it is known that LH is produced in large amounts while normal or decreased quantities of FSH are produced. There is also an increase in the production of insulin which is a hormone that helps the body to control the utilization of glucose. Insulin is produced by the pancreas. The need for increased insulin production arises because the patient's body tissues are not sensitive to the action of normal levels of insulin. This is called peripheral insulin resistance. Finally, the effective level of androgens such as testosterone in the body is higher than usual. Androgens are male hormones. The female normally produces a small amount of these hormones in her adrenal glands because they are needed for some of the activities that take place in her body. For example, androgens from the female adrenal glands help stimulate the growth of pubic and armpit hair. In polycystic ovary syndrome (PCOS) the ovaries also produce more androgens than normal. It is the high level of these androgens that makes some patients with PCOS have acne, greasy hair and excessive body hair. However, the level of androgens in these females is still not up to that

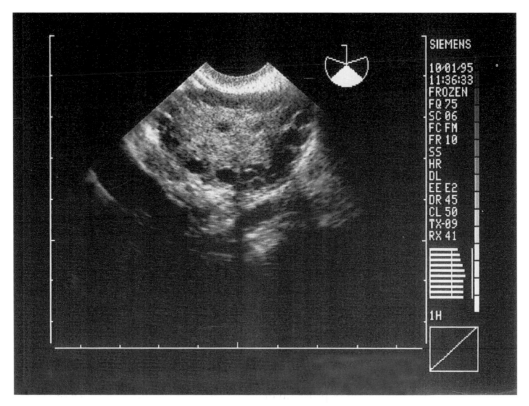

Figure 5.5   Transvaginal sonogram showing a polycystic ovary. Numerous follicular cysts are arranged around the periphery of the ovary giving a typical 'necklace' appearance.

normally found in men. Although obesity may not necessarily cause PCOS it worsens the problem. Obese PCOS patients who succeed in losing weight have an improvement of their symptoms and may ovulate spontaneously or in response to lower drug doses than previously. It is now being recognized that the hyperinsuli-naemia that is found in many women with PCOS induces changes in the body that lead to a wide range of potential problems in future. Such problems include dyslip-idaemia, atherosclerotic (coronary artery) heart disease, myocardial infarction, hypertension, glucose intolerance or non-insulin dependent diabetes, endometrial hyperplasia and endometrial cancer. Patients who succeed in becoming pregnant have a higher risk of miscarriage.

Weight loss

A female's body mass, especially the fat content, has an influence on her ovarian function. Menstruation does not commence until the body fat reaches a certain proportion of the total body mass. Even afterwards, regular ovulation and men-struation can only occur if the appropriate body fat content is maintained. Females who are underweight often cease to ovulate and to have menstrual periods. Although the reason for this is not too clear, it is known that FSH and LH secretion falls in such females and there is little or no development of ovarian follicles. Restoration of the normal body weight and fat content leads to a return of normal FSH and LH secretion, follicular development, ovulation and menstrual periods.

Strenuous exercise

Long distance female runners, gymnasts, ballet dancers and all those involved in intensive strenuous physical training tend to have problems with ovulation and menstruation similar to those described above. Although the present group of females may lose some weight during their training, weight loss is not invariable. The main cause of their ovulatory problems is the fact that they lose their fat stores such that the proportion remaining in the body falls below the critical level required for the maintenance of normal ovarian function.

Hyperprolactinaemia

Prolactin is one of the hormones that is produced by the pituitary gland. Its main function is to promote breast development during pregnancy in preparation for breast-feeding after delivery. It also stimulates the secretion of breast milk. The concentration of prolactin in the circulation is therefore high during pregnancy and lactation. High levels of prolactin in blood is given the name hyperprolactinaemia. It is normal in pregnancy and during breast-feeding but it is an abnormal finding at other times. Stress can lead to hyperprolactinaemia but the increase in hormone levels is short lived. However, if the prolactin level is found to be persistently high the pituitary gland is examined by X-ray photographs or using other imaging techniques such as CT (computed tomography) and MRI (magnetic resonance imaging) scans. This is because pituitary tumours are common causes of hyperprolactinaemia. These are benign (non-cancerous) tumours that can be very small (microadenoma) or larger (macroadenoma) in size and are called prolactinomas. Other benign tumours of the pituitary gland, hypothalamus or related organs, that do not produce prolactin, can still cause hyperprolactinaemia by interrupting the control pathways through which the hypothalamus inhibits the production of prolactin by the pituitary gland. Other causes of hyperprolactinaemia include certain medications such as metoclopramide, haloperidol, methyldopa, reserpine, thioxanthines and the phenothiazines. Drugs of abuse such as opiates and cocaine can have similar effects. Kidney, liver and thyroid dysfunction (hypothyroidism), head injury, brain infections and many other disorders may be implicated at times in the causation of hyperprolactinaemia. In some patients no cause is found for the elevated prolactin concentration. A few females with hyperprolactinaemia will continue having their menstrual periods. However, most others will cease to ovulate

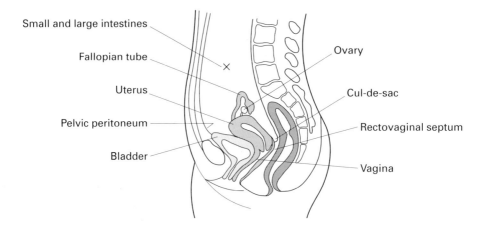

Small and large intestines

Fallopian tube

Uterus

Pelvic peritoneum

Bladder

Ovary

Cul-de-sac

Rectovaginal septum

Vagina

Figure 5.6   Sites of endometriosis in the pelvis.

and do not have menstrual periods. This is because hyperprolactinaemia interferes with the secretion of GnRH by the hypothalamus. Since there is no ovarian activity, the oestrogen levels in the female are quite low and they may suffer from dryness of the vagina and other menopause-type problems such as osteoporosis. Another symptom, which is not present in every patient, is that of unprovoked discharge of milk from the nipples, called galactorrhoea.

Endometriosis

Endometriosis is the name given to the condition in which tissue similar to the endometrium is found outside the uterine cavity. This is a common condition in certain parts of the world, especially in infertile women. Some have estimated that 20% of women have endometriosis at some stage in their lives. The endometriotic tissue can be found in various parts of the body but most commonly in the pelvis. The tissue may be found on the ovaries and tubes. It can also be found on the lining of the pelvic wall (called the peritoneum) (Figure 5.6). The reason why endometrium-like tissue exists outside the uterine cavity is not clear. Some theories have tried but do not provide a complete explanation for the appearance of this tissue in all reported sites. All that is known is that endometriosis is related in some way to menstruation. It is less common in females who start having children early or have many children. It is possible that the absence of menstrual periods during pregnancy and lactation allows the body enough time to tackle and eliminate any small area of developing endometriosis.

The problem with endometriotic tissue is that it responds to oestrogen and progesterone just like the endometrium that lines the uterine cavity. It therefore increases in thickness during the proliferative and secretory phases of the men-

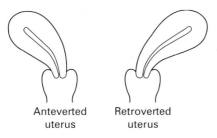

Anteverted   Retroverted
uterus   uterus

Figure 5.7   Diagrams depicting anteversion and retroversion of the uterus.

strual cycle and breaks down into pieces of tissue and blood during the time of menstruation. While the menstrual loss from the endometrium that lines the uterine cavity normally leaves the body through the cervical canal and vagina, the broken down tissue and blood from the endometriotic tissue in the pelvis and on the pelvic organs have nowhere to go. These irritate the peritoneum causing pain. The pain corresponds to the time of menstruation but is distinct from the 'period type pain' many women normally have. It tends to be more severe and lasts longer. Many have described it as a dull constant pain that is frequently felt in the back. Pain can also be felt at any other time during the menstrual cycle and during sexual intercourse. Surprisingly some women with endometriosis do not have any pain at all despite having large endometriotic deposits in the pelvis. Other symptoms of endometriosis include an increase in the amount of menstrual blood loss and the appearance of problems such as irregular periods.

The body responds to the presence of irritants in the pelvis by forming adhesions in an attempt to wall them off and prevent further irritation of the peritoneum. With each menstrual cycle more endometriotic tissue is formed, more irritant material accumulates in the pelvis and more adhesions result. There comes a time when the adhesions begin to involve part or all of the fallopian tubes and ovaries. In fact these adhesions can bury the tubes and ovaries such that ovulated oocytes cannot pass into the tube. Even in milder cases it is believed that the endometriotic tissue produces toxic compounds that can interfere with the interaction between the spermatozoa and oocyte in the fallopian tube thereby causing infertility. Endometriosis also interferes with ovulation in about 10% of patients. A formal system for classifying the severity of endometriosis was developed by the American Society for Reproductive Medicine. Generally the severity of endometriosis is graded as minimal, mild, moderate or severe.

Adhesions can hold the uterus in abnormal positions. The most common is the retroverted position. Here the uterus lies backwards instead of forwards like it normally does in most females (Figure 5.7). The problem is not in being retroverted since about 25% of women can have a retroverted uterus in the absence of endometriosis. Such women have normal fertility and their uterus can easily change from the retroverted to anteverted (falling forward) position. The problem in the retroversion that is found in endometriosis, and other conditions where adhesions form in the pelvis, is that the uterus is bound down in that position and cannot change to the anteverted position. This will not necessarily cause infertility unless the tubes and ovaries are also affected as described above. Fixed retroversion and the involvement of other parts of the pelvis including the vagina may make sexual intercourse very painful for these women. Tender nodules or lumps may be felt in the vaginal wall and surrounding areas during vaginal examination. The diagnosis and treatment of endometriosis in infertile couples will be considered in Chapters 6 and 7.

No detectable problem

There are females in whom no cause for the infertile condition is found even after detailed evaluation. The various techniques that are used for the evaluation of infertile couples are presented in Chapter 6. In summary the female must have a normal clinical history with no evidence of a sexual problem. Investigations should demonstrate normal midcycle cervical mucus with adequate penetration by spermatozoa and no evidence of cervical hostility. The uterus and uterine cavity must be deemed suitable for implantation. The tubes must be shown to be normal and open with the pelvis not showing any evidence of endometriosis or adhesions severe enough to impede conception. Finally the ovaries must be shown to ovulate regularly.

As can be seen from Figure 5.1, about 17% of females in infertile unions do not have a demonstrable problem to cause or contribute to their infertility. This proportion varies from region to region and also between hospitals. It is also true that the more extensive and complex the evaluation of the patient, the more problems that will be detected. However, many of the so-called fertility problems will also be found in women who have not had any difficulty in conceiving and having children. This makes some of these extra tests and their results unreliable because they cannot be used with confidence in planning a management strategy for the infertility. Furthermore, the tests are expensive, and some are invasive. They add unnecessary stress to an already difficult situation. Finally, these extra tests either do not provide any useful information for the management of a patient or they complicate the patient's problem further.

Conclusion

More is known about female factor problems than those of the male. This makes it easier to identify patients with obvious problems such as anovulation and tubal blockage, and to provide appropriate treatments. For the more nebulous problems, and females in whom no cause is found for the infertility, the decision to provide treatment and the particular treatment to give may depend more on factors that relate to age concerns and the couple's readiness to embark on treatment that may be expensive, than the nature of the infertility problem.

BIBLIOGRAPHY

Balen, A. H. & Jacobs, H. S. (1997). *Infertility In Practice.* New York: Churchill Livingstone.

Forman, R., Gilmour-White, S. & Forman, N. (1996). *Drug Induced Infertility and Sexual Dysfunction.* Cambridge: Cambridge University Press.

Insler, V. & Lunenfeld, B. (Eds) (1993). *Infertility: Male and Female,* 2nd edn. Edinburgh: Churchill Livingstone.

Kovacs G. (Ed.) (1997). *The Subfertility Handbook: A Clinician's Guide.* Cambridge: Cambridge University Press.

Meniru, G. I. & Akagbosu, F. T. (1997). Patient selection and management. In *A Handbook of Intrauterine Insemination,* ed. G. I. Meniru, P. R. Brinsden & I. L. Craft, pp. 23–45. Cambridge: Cambridge University Press.

Rebar, R. W. (1998). Assessment of the female patient. In *Textbook of Reproductive Medicine,* ed. B. R. Carr & R. E. Blackwell, 2nd edn, pp. 271–87. Stamford: Appleton & Lange.

Rowe, P. J., Comhaire, F. H., Hargreave, T. B. & Mellows, H. J. (1993). *WHO Manual for the Standardized Investigation and Diagnosis of the Infertile Couple.* Cambridge: Cambridge University Press.

Rowe, P. J., Comhaire, F. H., Hargreave, T. B. & Mahmoud, A. M. A. (2000). *WHO Manual for the Standardized Investigation, Diagnosis and Management of the Infertile Male.* Cambridge: Cambridge University Press.

Speroff, L., Glass, R. H. & Kase, N. G. (1999). Female Infertility. In: *Clinical Gynecologic Endocrinology and Infertility,* 6th edn, pp. 1013–42. Baltimore: Lippincott Williams & Wilkins.

Tan, S. L. & Jacobs, H. S. (1991). *Infertility: Your Questions Answered.* Singapore: McGraw-Hill Book Company.

Tindall, V. R. (1987). Malformations and maldevelopments of the genital tract. In *Jeffcoate's Principles of Gynaecology,* 5th edn, pp. 138–58. London: Butterworth & Co. (Publishers) Ltd.

6

Evaluation of the infertile couple

Introduction

There comes a time when a couple who have been trying unsuccessfully to start a family decide to seek medical attention. The timing of this decision varies; some may present to the clinician after just a few months of trying while others only do so after several years. There are no hard and fast rules about when to seek medical attention for infertility. On empirical grounds one can advise 12–18 months, knowing that it may take up to 12 months or so for the majority of couples to become pregnant naturally. Some clinicians may advocate a period of two years since spontaneous conceptions can and do still occur up till this time and even afterwards. However, such advice should take into consideration the individuals in question and factors such as the woman's age, the presence of symptoms suggesting an underlying cause for their infertility, whether the couple would wish to have infertility treatment at that time or whether they wish to wait for some more time before having any evaluation or treatment. For example, a 38-year-old female partner, in a couple who have been trying unsuccessfully for one year to have children, should be evaluated immediately because she does not have many more years remaining of optimal functioning of the ovaries. A couple who present with a history that is highly suggestive of a problem, such as persistently irregular menstrual periods or impotence, should also be evaluated immediately irrespective of how long they have been trying. In essence, although the statistics of natural conception are well known, one should never offer advice that bears no relationship to the particular case being considered. Furthermore, there is no way one can be sure that one or both partners of a couple do not have a significant infertility problem without performing some form of evaluation. Any couple who are sufficiently anxious to seek medical opinion should have at least a minimum of investigations capable of identifying any of the well known and unequivocal causes of infertility such as ovulatory dysfunction, blocked fallopian tubes and severe abnormality of the semen parameters. It is not humane that couples should have to wait for two years or more to discover they have any of these problems. If nothing else, early diagnosis will ensure the couple have more time available for treatment before advancing female age becomes an additional problem. Couples in whom no problem is detected or a mild abnormality found, for example, slight reduction in the concentration of spermatozoa, will be better disposed to try for natural conception a little while longer.

The most important step in the management of infertility is the evaluation of the couple to determine whether any cause for the condition can be found. It is only after this is completed that issues relating to treatment can be realistically discussed. It is recommended that both partners are seen at the same time. Neither of the partners in infertile couples can be assumed to be free of a cause for the problem. Each will have to be assessed using standard procedures. The discovery of a problem in one partner does not absolve the other from being properly assessed, as in about 20% or more of infertile couples both partners will have an identifiable problem. The evaluation of infertile couples is in four stages namely: clinical history, physical examination, routine infertility investigations and additional investigations.

The clinical history is obtained and physical examination carried out when the couple first present at the infertility clinic. Several questions are asked, aimed at finding out any obvious cause for the infertility. The World Health Organization (WHO) (Rowe et al., 1993, 2000) has provided a set of standard questions that infertile couples need to be asked and these will be adapted for the purposes of this chapter with additional questions being added. The questions are quite extensive and probe all aspects of each partner's social, medical and sexual life. In fact some couples may find some of the questions embarrassing but they are being asked in a constructive manner and seek to find the best way of helping the couple. It is important that couples are aware of the nature of these questions beforehand. Such foreknowledge assists greatly when the clinical history is being obtained at the clinic since the couple will have already had an opportunity to think about the questions and be more likely to give accurate responses with less waste of time. Both partners are examined at the clinic, following which they are scheduled for investigations. Further investigations may at times be required to clarify the significance and/or severity of detected problems.

Preliminary information from the couple

The clinical history of the couple starts with important biographical data which not only is important for administrative purposes but also helps in the management of the infertility. For example, the religious beliefs and ethnic origin/culture of the couple may determine the way they are evaluated, days they can have investigations and treatment. This could also exclude certain treatment options from consideration. The biographical information required from each partner includes surname, first name, date of birth, age, religion, ethnic group, citizenship and home address. It is important to establish very reliable communication links. The home, workplace and mobile telephone numbers, fax numbers and electronic mail address, if available, are recorded. Finally, the postal address is required. The couple should state how they wish to be contacted by the hospital and whether mail should be sent to them and which address to use. This is important because of the delicate nature of infertility and the fact that many couples may not have told their relatives and acquaintances of their seeking medical assistance. The next question that is normally asked is the duration of the infertility and whether the couple have had a pregnancy together in the past. Subsequently, the woman is evaluated followed by the man.

Evaluation of the female partner

Clinical history

The following information will be required from the female partner:
- Number and outcome of previous pregnancies in the present or previous marital union(s). The outcome of a pregnancy could be a viable birth, miscarriage, induced abortion, ectopic pregnancy or molar pregnancy.
- Number of living children.
- Any complications after delivery or miscarriage in the last pregnancy.
- Family planning methods used since the last pregnancy.
- Contraceptives that have ever been used if the female has never been pregnant.
- Previous investigation(s) for infertility.
- Previous treatment(s) for infertility.
- Diseases that may affect fertility such as diabetes, tuberculosis and thyroid disease.
- Medical treatment received for illness in the past. The clinician will be interested in medications such as cytotoxic (anticancer) drugs and so on.
- Operations such as appendectomy and gynaecological operations.
- Pelvic infection in the past.
- Sexually transmitted infections, for example, gonorrhoea and chlamydia.
- Abnormal (offensive or purulent) vaginal discharge.
- Galactorrhoea (discharge of milk) from the breast in a woman who is not breast-feeding or who has never been pregnant.
- Exposure of the woman to toxins in her home or work environment.
- Excessive alcohol consumption or drug abuse.
- Age at which the first menstrual period occurred.
- Regularity of the menstrual periods. Do they happen every 25–35 days?
- Length of the menstrual cycle (in days) (average, shortest and longest).

- Number of days in which she normally bleeds during each menstrual cycle (average, shortest and longest).
- Is the menstrual bleeding normal or abnormal in any way, for example, heavy and in clots?
- Pain during menstruation and its timing.
- Intermenstrual bleeding (bleeding at any other time of the cycle apart from when she normally has her menstrual periods).
- Post-coital bleeding (bleeding after sexual intercourse).
- First day of her last spontaneous menstrual period (day/month/year).
- Does the patient know how to determine her fertile period?
- If YES, has she tried timing sexual intercourse to take place at these fertile periods?
- How many times do the couple have sexual intercourse in a month.
- Has the pattern of sexual intercourse changed. Is the frequency of intercourse less, more or similar to what it was previously, or does intercourse only take place nowadays during the fertile period.
- Pain during sexual intercourse and where it is felt.

Physical examination

Just as in the clinical history, examination of the female is aimed at finding out if there are features that will point to a cause for the infertility. At the same time the woman is assessed for her suitability to have any of the infertility treatments and whether she is fit to have an operation involving general anaesthesia. The sequence of examination is usually as follows:

- General observation of the woman to gain an impression of her state of health.
- Height and weight measurement and calculation of the body mass index (BMI). The BMI is a way of assessing an individual's build to determine whether he or she is overweight, underweight or normal weight. It is derived by dividing the weight (in kilograms) by the square root of the height (in metres) i.e. $BMI = weight (kg)/height^2 (m)$. The BMI should ideally lie between 20–25. Values above this range indicate obesity while those below the range suggest underweight.
- Blood pressure measurement and checking the pulse. The clinician will also examine the chest to make sure the heart sounds and air entry into the lungs are normal. The findings made during this aspect of the examination relate more to the requirements for general anaesthesia than to the infertility itself.
- Assessment of body hair distribution. There should be a satisfactory growth of hair in the pubic region and armpit. Excessive growth of hair on the face and body may suggest the presence of polycystic ovary syndrome (PCOS) (see Chapter 5) although this is by no means invariable.

- Assessment of breast development. This should be normal. This is also an opportunity to examine the breasts to make sure there are no palpable tumours. The woman is encouraged to examine her breasts at regular intervals.
- Gentle squeezing of the nipples to see whether milky fluid can be expressed (galactorrhoea). The presence of galactorrhoea may mean that the patient has hyperprolactinaemia. However, fluid normally can be expressed from the nipples of women who have been pregnant and/or who have breast-fed before.
- Examination of the abdomen with a view to finding out if there are any tumours or tenderness. Abdominal tumours may be large uterine fibroids or ovarian tumours. Both have to be treated first before attempting to provide treatment for the infertility. Tenderness in the lower part of the abdomen may be due to pelvic infection. Scars from previous operations are sought for.
- Vaginal and pelvic examination to check on the state of the external genitalia, vagina, cervix and uterus. The ovaries usually cannot be felt unless they are enlarged. The presence of tumours in the pelvis is checked for. Any tenderness on pelvic examination is noted.

Routine investigations

The function of the reproductive organs and their associated organs can be assessed using a number of tests. A large range of tests are available but only those that are in common usage will be described. Some of the other tests will be mentioned for the sake of condemning their continued use.

Tests for ovulation

The only direct evidence that a female ovulates regularly is to observe the oocyte leaving the ovary at the moment of ovulation every month. However, this is not feasible since there is presently no method for observing the ovaries continuously without causing harm to the woman. Rather, indirect methods are used and they usually depend on the effects caused by events leading to ovulation and/or afterwards. When these effects are documented in a woman it can be assumed that ovulation has taken place. The common indices of ovulation and indirect methods are shown in Table 6.1.

Basal body temperature (BBT) monitoring
This test is based on the fact that post-ovulatory levels of progesterone raise the body temperature slightly (by about 0.5 °C). The woman checks her temperature with a thermometer everyday, usually before getting out of bed in the morning, and notes the reading on a chart. Following ovulation the corpus luteum begins to secrete progesterone and the thermometer should register a rise in the body temperature. This increase in temperature is usually maintained for about 10 days

Table 6.1. Methods of checking for the occurrence of ovulation

---

Basal body temperature monitoring
Cervical mucus changes
Endometrial biopsy
Ultrasonography of the ovaries and endometrium
Day 21 progesterone assay
Luteinizing hormone surge detection

---

before it falls to normal levels in those who do not become pregnant. The pattern that emerges when this temperature change is plotted on a graph during that month is said to be 'biphasic'. There are a number of problems with this method. The temperature measurement may not be accurate and will fluctuate depending on whether the female, for example, has a fever from some other cause or had been recently involved in physical activity. It may be difficult for the woman to interpret the readings she gets. The test does not tell the patient when ovulation is going to occur in future. It just tells her that ovulation probably occurred a day or two prior to the temperature rise. This information will not be useful to the couple who wish to have intercourse at the fertile part of the menstrual cycle because by the time the temperature is elevated the oocyte is likely not to be fertilizable. Furthermore, it does not necessarily mean that a woman whose chart does not show a temperature rise has not ovulated. In fact more than 50% of women with the so-called 'monophasic' pattern are found to ovulate regularly when more reliable tests are used to monitor ovulation. In summary, BBT measurement is not accurate, can be easily affected by other factors and does not predict the occurrence of ovulation. Most importantly it can increase the stress to which infertile couples are subjected. BBT is not advocated nowadays for these reasons.

Cervical mucus

Most females will notice that they have different types of vaginal secretions at various times during the menstrual cycle. As was described in Chapter 2 a distinctive type of mucus is produced by the cervical glands in the days preceding ovulation. This preovulatory mucus is clear in appearance, copious in amount and can be made to stretch over a distance of a few centimetres. Some women describe a slippery feeling in the vulva during that time period. Many will notice the mucus very often after passing urine and wiping themselves. Some may have to insert a finger slightly into the vagina to feel the mucus. Production of the preovulatory mucus as a result of the action of oestrogen is maximal just before ovulation. The mucus is noticed for two to three days before it disappears and is replaced by a scanty whitish secretion due to the action of progesterone on the cervical glands.

When a female notices this, it means that ovulation probably occurred within the past 24 hours or so.

Endometrial biopsy

A few strips of the endometrium can be removed by curettage on Days 24–27 of the cycle. This endometrial biopsy specimen is sent to the pathology laboratory where it is examined to determine if changes can be found in the structure of the tissue that indicate the action of progesterone on the endometrium as described in Chapter 2. If the expected secretory changes are found, it can be inferred that ovulation occurred about 10 days previously. This test is not commonly used nowadays since there are less invasive options. Normally, to obtain an endometrial biopsy specimen the patient is administered a general anaesthetic and the operation known as D & C (dilatation and curettage) performed. Endometrial biopsy can also be carried out in the outpatient clinic with the patient awake; smaller instruments and disposable thin plastic aspiration devices are used but it is frequently still a painful procedure, or at best uncomfortable, for the patient. These procedures are not innocuous. In addition to the discomfort, the uterus might be perforated accidentally with instruments that are inserted into it or infection introduced into the uterine cavity from where it may reach the pelvis and tubes causing tubal damage and pelvic adhesions. An undiagnosed pregnancy can also be interrupted. One of the very few indications for endometrial biopsy nowadays is the diagnosis of endometrial tuberculosis which is not very common, at least in the western world, although more common in some developing countries.

Ultrasonography of the ovaries and endometrium

Ovulation can be diagnosed by ultrasound scanning of the ovaries during the menstrual cycle. The actual ovulation is not observed. Rather the development of ovarian follicles is monitored by ultrasound, which is performed daily or every other day, towards the expected time of ovulation. Scanning is commenced in most cases from about Day 10. Normally the developing follicle appears round in shape and increases in size by about 2 mm a day in the latter part of the follicular phase. The follicle may reach a size of 22–24 mm or more prior to ovulation. Ovulation is taken to have occurred if the rounded appearance of the follicle disappears on a subsequent scanning episode. At this time the follicle appears collapsed and its walls are irregular in shape; this is when the corpus luteum begins to develop. Furthermore, there is evidence of a small amount of fluid in the pelvis and this usually comes from the follicle at the time of ovulation.

The endometrium can be examined with ultrasound during the menstrual cycle, because it increases in thickness during the proliferative and luteal phases. Additionally, it appears brighter in the latter part of the proliferative phase and this brightness is maximal during the luteal phase due to the action of progesterone. Again, it can be inferred that ovulation occurred in that cycle if such features are found. Ultrasound scanning for the prediction of ovulation is expensive and time consuming; it entails many hospital visits. It is not usually used routinely except in special cases. Ultrasound monitoring of follicular and endometrial development is mainly used during assisted conception treatments such as in vitro fertilization or ovulation induction.

Day 21 progesterone assay

This is the most cost effective method of documenting the occurrence of ovulation. A blood sample is withdrawn and analysed to measure the concentration of progesterone. This test is normally carried out on Day 21 of a menstrual cycle that normally lasts about 28 days. If however the menstrual cycle of a particular female regularly exceeds 28 days, say 35 days, the timing of the test can be adjusted to Day 28 of the cycle. In order words, the progesterone assay is carried out seven days before the expected commencement of the next menstrual period. Put another way, the test should be timed to take place about one week after ovulation. If the concentration of progesterone is found to be equal to or above 30 nmol/l it can be inferred that ovulation occurred in that cycle. When there is confusion regarding the menstrual cycle length of any particular patient, blood samples are withdrawn for the assay on two or three days spaced apart during the luteal phase of the cycle.

Luteinizing hormone surge detection

Another indirect method for assessing whether a female ovulates is the detection of the surge in luteinizing hormone (LH) production. The LH levels in the body can be monitored using blood tests. This is however, not a convenient method since frequent blood samples have to be withdrawn on a daily basis until the surge is detected. Fortunately, there are now ovulation predictor kits available in pharmacies that can be used to check urine samples for the appearance of the LH. The urine can be checked once or twice a day but to reduce costs the test can be carried out once a day. Since it is known that the LH surge normally starts after midnight, it is likely that testing the first urine sample produced after waking up in the morning will give the most accurate timing in this circumstance, but some manufacturers recommend testing the second urine sample of the day. However, some workers advocate testing the urine in the evening rather than morning. Ovulation normally occurs about 36 hours from the onset of the surge. Since the exact time of onset of the LH surge is not known it is more prudent to assume that ovulation will occur within 24 hours of the detection of LH in the early morning urine sample. The test is usually commenced about four days before the date of expected ovulation. For a 28-day cycle that means from Day 10. For a 35-day cycle that means Day 18.

Infertile couples can use this test kit to time intercourse more accurately to improve their chances of conception. It is probably the most convenient home monitoring method for predicting ovulation.

Other hormone tests

The concentration of follicle stimulating hormone (FSH) and LH can be measured by blood tests carried out on any of the following days of the cycle (Day 2, 3, 4 or 5) and provides useful information on the function of the ovaries. The FSH concentration is usually very high in women with failing ovaries. The LH concentration tends to be moderately elevated and is higher than that of FSH in women with PCOS. The FSH concentration in these women is usually normal. The concentration of androgens is elevated but not as high as levels found in males; any woman with higher levels should be evaluated to exclude androgen producing tumours. The concentration of both hormones is low in women with weight-loss or exercise induced ovulatory dysfunction. FSH and LH are almost undetectable in females with hypogonadotrophic hypogonadism.

Oestrogen levels can also be measured. The exact value depends on the part of the cycle in which it is measured. The result may be helpful in the diagnosis of certain ovulatory problems. A low oestrogen level suggests poor ovarian function such as is found in ovarian failure or in hypogonadotrophic hypogonadism.

The concentration of prolactin is also measured using a blood sample withdrawn on Day 2, 3, 4 or 5. If it is found to be high another sample of blood is withdrawn and the test repeated avoiding stress provoking actions since stress transiently increases the level of this hormone. Persistent elevation of the level of prolactin (hyperprolactinaemia) interferes with ovulation. Imaging of the brain by plain X-ray or preferably, MRI or CT scanning should be performed in patients with hyperprolactinaemia to determine if it is due to the presence of a tumour (called prolactinoma or adenoma) in the pituitary gland.

The function of the thyroid gland is assessed by measuring the concentration of thyroid stimulating hormone, thyroxine and tri-iodotyronine in blood. In most instances this will be normal but it is still a useful screening test because of the occasional patient who has unrecognized thyroid gland dysfunction.

Tubal patency tests

Rubin's test

This test is being mentioned just to condemn its continued usage. It involves passing carbon dioxide gas through the cervix and listening with a stethoscope for the sound of gas bubbling through the open ends of the fallopian tubes and into the pelvis. This test is very inaccurate and has no place in the evaluation of infertile couples.

Hysterosalpingogram (HSG)

HSG is a special X-ray photograph showing the outline of the uterine cavity and the two fallopian tubes. The procedure (hysterosalpingography a.k.a. HSG) is used to determine whether a woman's tubes are open or blocked. It will also show whether there is alteration of the shape of the uterine cavity by tumours such as fibroids or whether there is a uterine malformation. It is also useful in the diagnosis of Asherman's syndrome. The test is normally performed when the woman is most likely not to be pregnant. This is usually within the first 10 days of the menstrual cycle. The menstrual bleeding may last for three days in some women, and up to seven days in others. The HSG is not carried out while the bleeding is still present. It should be performed anytime after the bleeding stops.

A gown is usually provided by the hospital for the patient to wear during the test to avoid soiling or rumpling her own clothes. She lies down on a special table in the X-ray room and a speculum is gently inserted into the vagina to allow the cervix to be seen. The speculum is similar to the one that is used when a cervical smear (pap smear) is being performed. The cervix is wiped clean of secretions and a pair of forceps clipped onto it. A cannula is then attached to the cervix; this is a tube through which the X-ray dye is injected into the uterus. There are different types of cannulas but they serve the same function.

The gynaecologist will slowly inject the special X-ray dye using the cannula. The radiologist will take photographs as the dye flows up the uterine cavity and through the fallopian tubes. If the tubes are open the dye will also spill out of the fallopian tubes and into the pelvis. A sample of HSG findings are shown in Figures 6.1–6.3.

Women have described their experience of HSG in different ways. Some say that it is 'just a little bit uncomfortable' whilst others say that it is painful. It appears that the major sensation felt during the test is that of uterine cramps similar to the cramps that occur during the menstrual period. The most important thing to bear in mind is that the unpleasant part of the test does not last long (maximum 30 seconds). To decrease any discomfort or pain felt at HSG, a non-steroidal anti-inflammatory drug is taken one to two hours beforehand. The discomfort will be less if the dye is injected slowly. Apart from this, no other preparation is needed. The patient rests for a short while before going home. She is advised to come with someone who will drive her home. She should not go back to work on that same day. The results of the test will be discussed at the next clinic attendance.

The patient should not be pregnant at the time of the test. If there is a previous history of pelvic infection another test such as laparoscopy and dye test should be performed instead. A history of allergy to iodine makes HSG unsafe because the X-ray dye that is used contains iodine. HSG should not be performed if the patient is bleeding. Problems are rarely associated with HSG. However, there is a chance of causing pelvic infection. There may be an allergic reaction to the iodine-containing

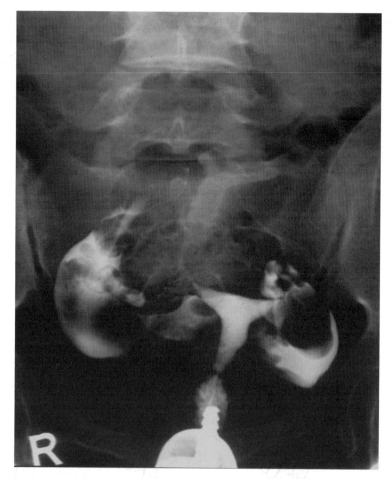

Figure 6.1   Hysterosalpingogram: spillage of contrast medium from the fimbrial end of both fallopian tubes indicating bilateral tubal patency.

X-ray dye. A vasovagal reflex may be triggered by cannulation of the cervix, especially in nulliparous patients leading to collapse, sweating, faintness and breathlessness.

HSG is an inexpensive and convenient screening test. It identifies a large proportion of women with tubal blockage. However, a laparoscopy and dye test is often required to confirm the findings made with the HSG. The HSG will not reveal any problems outside the fallopian tubes in the pelvis that may cause infertility such as endometriosis or adhesion formation from a previous pelvic infection. Unfortunately, the laparoscopy and dye test is a more expensive and inconvenient test than HSG, but the HSG still has a role in infertility investigations and the laparoscopy and dye test actually compliments HSG.

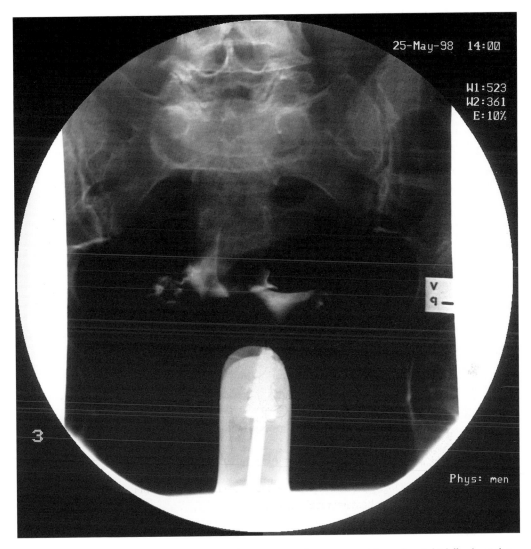

Figure 6.2   Hysterosalpingogram: spillage of contrast medium occurred from the right fallopian tube but not from the left tube. The left fallopian tube is only filled by contrast medium up the isthmic portion. Subsequent laparoscopy and dye test revealed both tubes to be patent and the pelvis free of stigmata of previous infection.

HyCoSy

This is a relatively new test of tubal patency that is somewhat similar to HSG but does not involve the use of X-rays. Instead the ultrasound scanner is used to monitor the flow of a specially compounded fluid medium that is slowly injected into the uterine cavity and fallopian tubes through the cervical canal. Ultrasound scanning is performed using a probe that is placed in the vagina. If the tubes are not

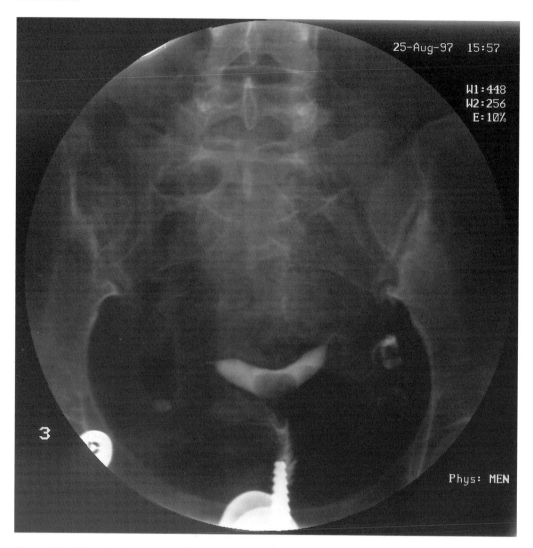

Figure 6.3 Hysterosalpingogram: bicornuate uterus.

blocked the fluid should be seen flowing through them. HyCoSy stands for hyster-osalpingo contrast sonography. It is still being evaluated but is not likely to be more accurate than HSG. It also suffers from a drawback similar to that of HSG in that the pelvis cannot be visualized. Therefore it cannot exclude the presence of adhesions in the pelvis even if the tubes are shown to be open.

Laparoscopy and dye test
Whenever possible, a laparoscopy and dye test should performed. This serves the dual purpose of checking for patency of the fallopian tubes as well as providing an

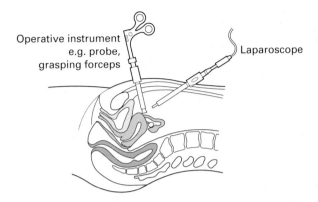

Operative instrument
e.g. probe,
grasping forceps

Laparoscope

Figure 6.4   Laparoscopy.

opportunity for the pelvis to be examined carefully to diagnose or exclude the presence of endometriosis, adhesions or any other problems that may be causing or contributing to the infertility. If performed in the luteal phase of the menstrual cycle it permits confirmation of ovulation in that cycle by observing the corpus luteum in the ovary, but care should be taken to ensure that the woman is not pregnant in that cycle. The couple are asked to use barrier contraceptives such as condoms or abstain from sex during the fertile period of that cycle.

Laparoscopy and dye test is usually performed as a day-case procedure. The patient comes to the hospital on the morning of the procedure having taken no food or fluid after the preceding midnight. She should be accompanied by her partner or any adult relative or friend. This is more important for after the procedure when she will need someone to drive her home or accompany her if she has to use the public transport system. Laparoscopy is normally carried out under general anaesthesia. The drugs that are used are short lasting and full consciousness is regained within a short while of completing the procedure. It is also possible for the laparoscopy to be performed under local anaesthesia with the patient sedated.

After establishing adequate anaesthesia a needle (called the *Verres* needle) is pushed through the abdominal wall into the abdominal cavity. About 1.5 litres of carbon dioxide gas are introduced through this needle into the abdomen to distend it and allow easy visualization of the pelvic organs. A small (~1 cm) elliptical incision is made just below the umbilicus. A laparoscope is inserted into the abdomen through this incision and used to inspect the ovaries, tubes and uterus (Figure 6.4). The pelvis itself is also inspected carefully looking for evidence of endometriosis and adhesions. Another incision is made lower down the abdomen for the introduction of instruments that are used in manoeuvring the pelvic organs around to permit their complete examination.

The dye test is carried out with the laparoscope still positioned in the abdomen.

A cannula is connected to the cervical canal and methylene blue dye is slowly injected. If the tubes are not blocked the blue dye will distend the tubes and then flow out of the open end of the fallopian tubes.

Afterwards, as much of the carbon dioxide gas as possible is removed from the abdomen and the small incision(s) closed with one or two sutures. The patient is allowed home accompanied, after resting for some hours. She should rest at home for a few days (two to three days) before resuming work. Laparoscopy is relatively safe but a number of complications are possible although uncommon. The woman may feel slightly bloated and uncomfortable but this settles within a day or so. Any of the abdominal or pelvic organs, including bowel and blood vessels, can be traumatized during the procedure. If the damage is substantial, a formal operating procedure may be required for the repair of the traumatized organ and the patient will need to be in hospital longer than anticipated. Some of the carbon dioxide gas may enter the blood stream as gas bubbles and reach the heart and lungs before being completely dissolved in the blood. This is called embolism and it is a desperate emergency condition. Embolism is not common with carbon dioxide; it is more common when other gases such as room air or nitrogen are used in place of carbon dioxide for laparoscopy.

Not all the carbon dioxide gas can be evacuated from the abdominal cavity after laparoscopy; the remaining gas will be slowly absorbed by the body and this may take up to a day or more for this to happen. During that time the gas tends to track upwards to the underside of the diaphragm whenever the patients sits or stands and irritate it; because of the origin of the nerve supply to the diaphragm the irritation may be felt as shoulder tip pain. The pain is however, self-limiting and will eventually subside. Another complication is that of carrying out laparoscopy and dye test in the presence of an early pregnancy. This is an uncommon complication and there is not much information on what happens to that pregnancy but it seems that it usually continues without problems. Couples must use barrier contraceptives for sexual intercourse or abstain completely in the month the woman has this procedure. A pregnancy test is necessary if the last menstrual period was not as expected and there is suspicion that the patient is already pregnant before the operative procedure.

Cervical mucus tests

There are a number of investigations that are based on the use of cervical mucus (Table 6.2), but they have not been popular or widely used by clinicians during evaluation of infertile couples. There are many reasons for this but the most common is the fact that there has not been adequate standardization of the techniques used for the tests; several clinicians and researchers use different modifications of the techniques. This might be the reason behind the inconsistent results

Table 6.2. Investigating the interaction between spermatozoa and cervical mucus

Post-coital test
The slide test
Sperm–cervical–mucus contact test
The capillary tube test

that have been obtained by different researchers who have tried to determine how best to use the tests in the management of infertility.

The most common is the post-coital test. The couple are asked to have intercourse at the middle of the cycle when production of the preovulatory mucus is supposed to be at its height. Intercourse is timed to occur late at night. The woman comes to the hospital the next morning without douching and a sample of mucus is gently withdrawn from the cervical canal using a special syringe or mucus collector. The interval between sexual intercourse and the test is usually 6–12 hours although some hospitals perform the test sooner while others carry it out later. The mucus is checked to see whether it can stretch into a thread which can be more than 5 cm long. This phenomenon is called spinnbarkheit. The volume of the mucus is also measured and the pH determined. Some of the mucus sample is placed on a glass slide and examined under the microscope. An adequate number of spermatozoa should be seen in the mucus moving rapidly in a straight line. The presence of cells such as white blood cells is checked for and their number estimated. All the various observations are computed into a result which, simply put, is either normal or abnormal.

A normal test suggests that spermatozoa can enter the cervical canal and move through the cervical mucus in which they survive for long periods. This means that the cervical mucus is not hostile to spermatozoa and is not the cause for the existing infertility. An abnormal test however does not mean that there is a problem. It may result from an improperly timed test, the test being performed at the time of the cycle when production of the preovulatory mucus has not yet commenced or has stopped. To avoid this, the woman should closely monitor her vaginal secretions towards the midpoint of the menstrual cycle and have the post-coital test performed on the second day of the appearance of the mucus. Surprisingly, an abnormal test can also mean that there was no sexual intercourse, no ejaculation or no ejaculation inside the vagina. In the absence of any of these as a cause for the abnormal test it is still difficult to make conclusive statements on the relevance of the abnormal post-coital test to the couple's infertility although a further search could be made to identify any of the causes of hostile cervical mucus mentioned in Chapter 5.

Optional investigations

Pelvic ultrasound scan

The ultrasound scanner can be regarded as an extension of the clinician's senses and assists him or her in improving the detection rate of problems that can have an influence on the welfare of patients. The technology of ultrasonography has been so refined that good quality images are now obtained and it is much easier to use. Ultrasound has revolutionized the management of infertility and, as will be seen in later chapters, it is an indispensable tool in the treatment of infertility especially using assisted conception methods. If possible, a patient should have an ultrasound scan at the stage of investigation of infertility. It will assist in the diagnosis of a wide range of infertility-associated pathology such as uterine malformations, fibroids, endometriotic cysts, polycystic ovaries and hydrosalpinges. It will also provide baseline information such as the size of the uterus and ovaries and allow the thickness and reflectivity of the endometrium to be measured.

Ultrasound scanning of the pelvic organs can be carried out with probes placed on the abdomen or in the vagina. A full bladder is required for the abdominal approach since this straightens out the uterus and moves it upwards so as to be nearer the ultrasound probe placed on the anterior abdominal wall. The woman is asked to drink a lot of fluid (up to one litre) two to three hours before the appointment and not to empty her bladder during that time. This can be quite uncomfortable. A full bladder is not required for the transvaginal approach. The transducer is covered with a fresh disposable rubber sheath to prevent cross-infection. It is gently introduced into the vagina and the pelvic organs are usually seen clearly on the screen. There are certain situations where the abdominal approach is preferred and others where the transvaginal approach is better.

Hysteroscopy

A hysteroscope can be described as a smaller version of the laparoscope which is used to view the uterine cavity. The hysteroscope is introduced through the cervical canal (Figure 6.5) and is useful in the diagnosis of uterine polyps, fibroids or malformations, Asherman's syndrome and some causes of abnormal uterine bleeding. A small amount of fluid or carbon dioxide is used to open up the uterine cavity to allow good vision during the procedure. Some operations can now be carried out inside the uterus using the hysteroscope including some assisted conception treatments. Hysteroscopy is performed as an outpatient procedure either in the clinic or theatre. For the clinic based procedure the patient may remain awake and have local anaesthesia and some sedation. In the theatre, hysteroscopy can be combined with the laparoscopy and dye test.

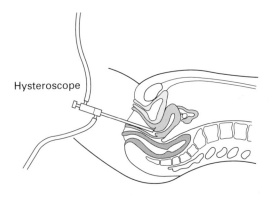

Hysteroscope

Figure 6.5 Hysteroscopy.

Other tests not related to the causes of infertility

There are some other tests that are carried out in infertile couples that are not strictly required for the diagnosis of the infertility.

A blood sample is taken to find out if the woman is immune to rubella (German measles). Rubella is a mild febrile illness in the adult and rashes appear later on in the disease process. These rashes disappear and the individual recovers completely becoming immune to further attacks. The situation is different if the woman happens to be pregnant and if she catches the infection in the first 12 weeks of the pregnancy. The virus will attack the fetus and cause severe malformations. For non-immune females a single injection of the vaccine will make them immune to rubella before they become pregnant. This is why infertile women are screened for immunity to rubella since it will indeed be a calamity if infertility is treated successfully only for the patient to contract rubella infection during pregnancy and have a malformed baby.

The infertility clinic is one of the health care settings where opportunistic screening for cervical cancer is carried out. Most centres will want to screen the patients for the human immunodeficiency virus (HIV) and for the hepatitis B and C viruses.

Other routine investigations will include blood grouping, full blood counts, urine tests and tests for sickle cell anaemia and thalassaemia in susceptible ethnic groups.

Additional investigations

Other tests not so far mentioned include measurement of androgen concentrations in blood in patients with PCOS or excessive body hair and tests for infections such as chlamydia in women with pelvic infection or sequalae such as blocked tubes or adhesions. These and other tests may be required to clarify a diagnosis and help in the treatment of the patient. They are however, not applicable to every female with infertility.

Female diagnosis

The WHO (Rowe et al., 1993) has proposed diagnostic categories for females evaluated for infertility. This is a functional classification that was designed with the purpose of positively assisting the management of these patients. By placing every evaluated patient in one of the following categories it is usually possible to decide whether any treatment is possible or needed and how it can be applied. The following adapted categories should be studied in conjunction with the female factor problems presented in Chapter 5.

- Sexual dysfunction.
- Hyperprolactinaemia.
- Organic lesions of the hypothalamus and pituitary region.
- Amenorrhoea (cessation of the menstrual periods for over six months) with elevated FSH.
- Amenorrhoea with adequate oestrogen levels in the body.
- Amenorrhoea with low oestrogen levels in the body.
- Oligomenorrhoea (intervals between periods greater than six weeks but less than six months).
- Irregular menses and/or ovulation.
- Anovulation with regular cycles.
- Congenital abnormalities.
- Blockage of both fallopian tubes.
- Pelvic adhesions.
- Endometriosis.
- Acquired uterine or cervical lesions.
- Acquired tubal lesions.
- Acquired ovarian lesions.
- Genital tuberculosis.
- Iatrogenic causes (causes arising from medical intervention such as formation of adhesions in the pelvis after pelvic surgery).
- Systemic causes such as diabetes and thyroid disease.
- Diagnosis not established because laparoscopy was not carried out. Laparoscopy is required to exclude pelvic pathology such as endometriosis and adhesions. A female cannot be said to be free of detectable causes of infertility without laparoscopy.
- Abnormal post-coital test.
- No demonstrable cause even after laparoscopy.

Evaluation of the male partner

Clinical history

Questions similar to the following are usually asked of the male partner.

- Has he made any woman pregnant before, even if the pregnancy did not result in a child.
- Previous investigation(s) for infertility.
- Previous treatment(s) for infertility.
- Medical disease such as diabetes, tuberculosis, chronic respiratory tract disease, fibrocystic disease of the pancreas, neurologic disease or other medical problems that may impair a man's fertility.
- Medical treatments of importance including the chronic use of drugs such as sulphasalazine or calcium channel blockers.
- High fever within the past six months.
- Genital operations such as repair of urethral strictures, hypospadias or inguinal hernia, prostatectomy, bladder neck surgery, vasectomy, hydrocoelectomy or sympathectomy. These operations can cause blockage of the male reproductive tract, retrograde ejaculation or anejaculation (lack of ejaculation).
- Urinary tract infection (cystitis, pyelonephritis)
- Sexually transmitted infections such as syphilis, gonorrhoea and chlamydia.
- Epididymitis (infection of the epididymides).
- Problems that can cause damage to the testes such as mumps, other infections, injury or torsion. In the last problem, the testis twists on its cord thereby shutting off its blood supply. If this is not rapidly relieved by an operation the torsion will lead to permanent damage to the testis.
- Varicocoele.
- Undescended testis that was either treated in childhood or is still persisting.
- The man's occupation and whether it has any impact on his fertility. Occupations in which the testes are exposed to temperatures that are higher than normal for long periods. This may include some types of office work in which the man sits down with thighs held close together for long periods, long distance truck drivers and furnace workers. Any deleterious effects are likely to be more pronounced in men who already have borderline abnormal semen parameters. Some occupations involve the use of chemicals that are toxic to the testes.
- Excessive consumption of alcohol.
- Smoking and number of cigarettes smoked per day.
- Drug abuse.
- Average frequency of intercourse per month.
- Is erection of the penis normal or inadequate?
- Is ejaculation normal or inadequate?

Physical examination

It is recommended that the male partner is examined during the clinic consultation because this may reveal abnormalities of importance such as varicocoele. The man should put on a loose examination gown and remain standing for 5–15 minutes before examination of the genitalia is performed. This manoeuvre may make scrotal swellings and varicocoeles become more prominent. The examination room should be maintained at 20–22 °C. The physical examination will encompass:

- Observation of the man's general appearance to gain an impression of his state of health.
- Height in metres.
- Weight in kilograms.
- Blood pressure measurement and the pulse.
- General physical examination including the chest (heart sounds and air entry into the lungs) and abdomen.
- A check for signs of normal virilization such as deepening of the voice, moustache, beard, armpit and pubic hair, size of the penis and testes.
- Any abnormalities of the penis, testes, epididymides and vasa deferentia.
- Specifically check for varicocoele, hydrocoele and inguinal hernia.
- Scars or swellings on the groin.
- Examination of the prostate and seminal vesicles. A gloved, lubricated finger is introduced into the rectum and used in palpating the prostate gland and seminal vesicles.

Investigations: semen analysis

This is the main laboratory investigation for the assessment of the male fertility potential. A sample of semen is examined in the laboratory checking several well defined parameters. These parameters together give a reasonably accurate impression of how normal the semen is. However, there has been great difficulty in defining the optimal value of these parameters. This is because some patients with relatively poor semen parameters can still father children provided their partner's fertility potential is high.

A semen sample is produced for analysis by masturbation after two to five days of abstinence from ejaculation. Usually an abstinence period of two to three days is adequate. This period of abstinence is for the purpose of standardization so that results from different men can be compared easily. The ejaculate is collected into sterile plastic containers that are non-toxic to spermatozoa. It is recommended that the man washes his hands and genitals with soap, rinses them several times with clean water and dries with a clean towel. No lubricant such as petroleum jelly is allowed during masturbation since most of these lubricants have been shown to be toxic to spermatozoa.

Although it is preferable to produce this sample within the hospital premises it is realized that some men may find it difficult masturbating on demand in strange environments. Such people can produce the sample at home and bring it in immediately. The sample should reach the laboratory within 30–60 minutes of production. Care should be taken to keep it warm. It, however, should not rest on domestic heaters since the spermatozoa will die immediately. The container can be carried in a shirt pocket close to the skin in cold climates. In warm climates, hot areas should be avoided. Again the sample is carried on the person and taken to the laboratory as soon as possible.

Rooms are specially set aside in fertility centres or laboratories for production of semen samples by masturbation. Such rooms are ideally located in a quiet part of the unit and a DO NOT DISTURB sign is hung on the door. Suitable magazines and video recordings are normally provided in these rooms for those who require them. Some men may find it impossible to masturbate because of psychological reasons. Such men are provided with special condoms to use during sexual intercourse. These are not the usual condoms that are available in shops and supermarkets that contain chemicals which kill spermatozoa. Semen collection condoms are made of silicone rubber material, which has been found not to be toxic to spermatozoa. Following ejaculation they are carefully removed from the penis and the semen emptied into the sterile jar that is provided.

Semen can be collected as whole or split ejaculate. In the first type the whole of the ejaculate is collected in one container and analysed as such. In the second type, the man is given two containers that are held together with adhesive tape. One of the containers is labelled as '1' while the other is labelled '2'. The man is instructed to commence ejaculating into Pot 1 and, after the first two spurts, to move to Pot 2 where he is to finish the ejaculation. The reason for this method of collection is that most of the ejaculated spermatozoa will be found in the first one or two spurts while the remaining part of the ejaculate consist of fluid from the various accessory organs. The samples in the two pots are analysed separately and the results combined. Split ejaculate is required by some fertility units while others use whole ejaculates for analysis and assisted conception treatments.

The constituents of semen have been described in earlier chapters. The technique of semen analysis is beyond the scope of the present book but details can be found both in the WHO (1992, 1999) manuals and the book on intrauterine insemination (Meniru et al., 1997). The WHO has provided the minimum values to be accepted as normal (Table 6.3). This does not mean that men with lower values cannot father children. They are given as guidelines only. However, it has been shown that the more abnormal a semen analysis result is, the more difficult it is for the man to establish a pregnancy naturally. There is no lower limit below which natural paternity is impossible except in cases where no spermatozoa is present in

Table 6.3. Normal values of standard semen analysis

Liquefaction	Complete within 60 minutes at room temperature
Appearance	Homogenous, grey opalescent
Odour	'fresh' and characteristic
Consistency	Leaves pipette as discrete droplets
Volume	2.0 ml or more
pH	7.2 or more
Sperm concentration	20×10^6 spermatozoa/ml or more
Total sperm count	40×10^6 spermatozoa per ejaculate or more
Motility	50% or more spermatozoa with forward progression (grades 'a' and 'b') or 25% or more with rapid linear progression (grade 'a') within 60 minutes of ejaculation
Morphology	30% or more spermatozoa with normal forms
Vitality	75% or more live spermatozoa
White blood cells	Fewer than 1×10^6/ml
Immunobead test	Fewer than 50% motile spermatozoa with beads bound
MAR test	Fewer than 50% motile spermatozoa with adherent particles

Source: World Health Organization (1992, 1999).

the ejaculate or all of them are dead. The following is a simplified description of the WHO normal values of semen analysis as outlined in Table 6.3.

Semen forms a clot immediately on ejaculation but this liquefies over the ensuing minutes and the process is usually complete within 30 minutes. Following liquefaction semen can easily be drawn into a pipette but some individuals produce semen that is viscous. One way of assessing viscosity is to allow the semen to leave a pipette slowly. Non-viscous samples will leave as discrete drops while viscous samples tend to flow out of the pipette as an unbroken thread of semen (Figure 6.6). The relevance of viscous semen to fertility has yet to be ascertained. Many fertile men have viscous semen but the speed of movement of spermatozoa is slowed down until they escape from the semen and into the cervical canal. Semen appears opalescent and is usually greyish-white but some samples look yellowish in colour. This may be because of a high intake of carotene in the diet. Carotene is utilized by the body to produce vitamin A and is found in high quantities in carrot and palm oil. The odour of semen is a little hard to describe and most people will just say that the odour is characteristic! Semen should however not have a foul odour.

About 2–6 ml of semen is produced by ejaculation. Higher volumes, such as 24 ml, have been produced. Semen is usually alkaline. The normal pH range was originally stated as 7.2–8.0 by the WHO (1992) but values of up to 8.5 have been noted

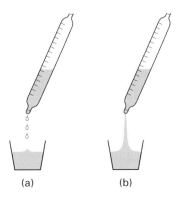

(a)   (b)

Figure 6.6   The viscosity of a semen sample can be assessed by observing how the sample flows out of a partially vented plastic pipette: (a) non-viscous semen will leave the pipette as discrete drops; while (b) semen of increased viscosity will flow out as an unbroken thread.

in apparently normal semen samples. There is no upper limit to the pH in the latest WHO publication (1999). The normal concentration of spermatozoa in the ejaculate should be 20 million/ml or more. This is an arbitrary cut-off point but there is a tendency for natural conception rates to decrease when the concentration falls below this value. About 50% or more of the spermatozoa in the ejaculate should be moving forward. The WHO defined four types of motility pattern which are named a, b, c and d. The 'a' type motility is the most desirable type and 25% or more of the spermatozoa must have this motility for the semen sample to be classified as being normal in that context. The 'a' type motility pattern is defined as rapid progressive motility, while the 'b' type is slow or sluggish progressive motility, the 'c' type is nonprogressive motility and the 'd' type is immotility.

All semen samples contain a significant proportion of spermatozoa with abnormal shapes. This is a normal finding even in the most fertile of men. The WHO (1992) stated that if 30% or more spermatozoa are normal in shape then the morphology score of the semen sample is normal. Since that recommendation was made several reports have shown that normal sperm morphology counts as low as 15% can be accepted as being normal. Although several spermatozoa may be stationary when observed under the microscope many of them are still living. In fact if observed long enough, previously stationary spermatozoa may start moving again. When a special dye (eosin–nigrosin dye) is mixed with a drop of the semen sample, dead spermatozoa will be stained pink and can be counted. It will then be possible to get a more accurate estimate of the proportion of live spermatozoa in the sample; the WHO says that it should be 75% or more. A white blood cell count higher than 1 million/ml suggests the presence of an infection but most times no infectious organism will be identified. The immunobead and

MAR tests check for the presence of antisperm antibodies in the semen sample. When antisperm antibodies are present a large proportion of spermatozoa will bind to the reagent particles and will be seen clearly under the microscope.

The parameters of each semen sample vary from those of other samples produced by the same individual often by significant values. This is why it is important to perform semen analysis on more than one sample produced by the same man at intervals of a few weeks or months. This is especially important when poor results are obtained in order to find out if that was a transient occurrence or a permanent feature of the individual's semen. From experience, poor semen samples do not really improve that much unless an episode of fever or severe illness occurred during production of the spermatozoa 74 days previously but was treated successfully afterwards. Poor quality semen resulting from the effects of cytotoxic drugs on the testes, may recover progressively over the months and years following cessation of treatment in some cases.

Additional investigations

The finding of an abnormality during history taking, physical examination or semen analysis may dictate the performance of additional investigations to shed further light on the problem and help decide on how to treat it if possible. The following tests may be required:

- Contact thermography and doppler ultrasound for varicocoele.
- Prostatic expression fluid and/or urine after prostatic massage for the diagnosis of infections of the prostate gland.
- Analysis of post-orgasm urine to identify spermatozoa in men suspected of having retrograde ejaculation.
- Measuring the concentration of hormones such as FSH, LH, prolactin and androgens in cases of severe abnormality of semen parameters including azoospermia.
- Special X-ray photographs (plain X-ray, MRI or CT scanning) of the brain performed in cases of hyperprolactinaemia (also in males!) to find out if it is being caused by pituitary tumours.
- Testicular biopsy in cases of azoospermia or severe oligozoospermia. A piece of testicular tissue is surgically removed, processed in the laboratory and examined under the microscope for signs of sperm production.

Other tests

- Screening for HIV and hepatitis B and C viruses.
- Blood group, full blood counts, analysis of urine and tests for sickle cell anaemia and thalassaemia in susceptible ethnic groups.
- Screening for abnormalities in the structure or number of the sex chromosomes and autosomes such as Y chromosome microdeletions (Rowe et al., 2000).

The male diagnosis

It is usually possible to assign the man to one of the following WHO diagnostic categories at the end of his evaluation.

- Sexual and/or ejaculatory problems.
- Immunological causes (antisperm antibodies detected in the man's semen or blood).
- No demonstrable cause.
- Isolated seminal plasma abnormalities (relates to the various compounds normally found in semen and are produced by the accessory sex glands).
- Iatrogenic causes (arising as complication of treatment such as blockage of vasa deferentia following inguinal hernia repair).
- Systemic causes such as high fever and some diseases.
- Congenital abnormalities such as severe hypospadias or undescended testes.
- Acquired testicular damage, for example, following mumps infection of the testes in adulthood.
- Varicocoele.
- Male accessory gland infection.
- Endocrine causes such as hypogonadotrophic hypogonadism.
- Idiopathic oligozoospermia.
- Idiopathic asthenozoospermia.
- Idiopathic teratozoospermia.
- Obstructive azoospermia, for example, in cases of congenital absence of both vasa deferentia or following vasectomy.
- Idiopathic azoospermia.

Conclusion

Evaluation of the infertile couple is the most crucial aspect of their management. If it is carried out efficiently and in an informed manner it is likely that subsequent management will be conducted in a similar manner thereby increasing the chances of successful treatment. The tests described here are as currently recommended by most fertility professional groups and other international bodies as necessary for the initial evaluation of the infertile couple. There are still several tests that have not been described such as computer assisted semen analysis (CASA) and the so-called sperm function tests; most are still at the research stage and do not at present contribute much to the initial decision-making process. Their description is not within the scope of this book. An unfortunate aspect of infertility management is still that of time wasting. Most couples spend a very long time being investigated and re-investigated in non-specialized health establishments. Yet it is possible to complete all basic infertility investigations within one month as shown in Figure 6.7. This chapter stresses the importance of a speedy diagnosis since it allows the couple

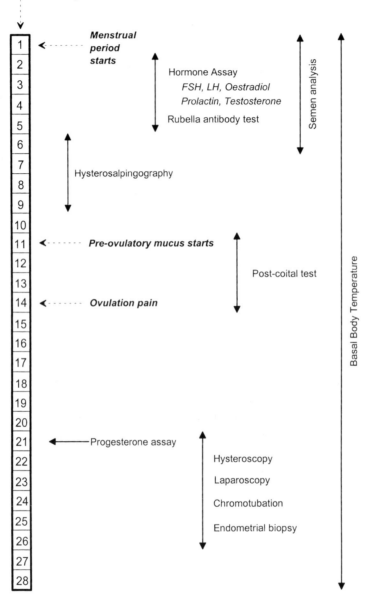

Figure 6.7   A scheme for the efficient investigation of infertile couples. Adapted from Meniru et al. (1997).

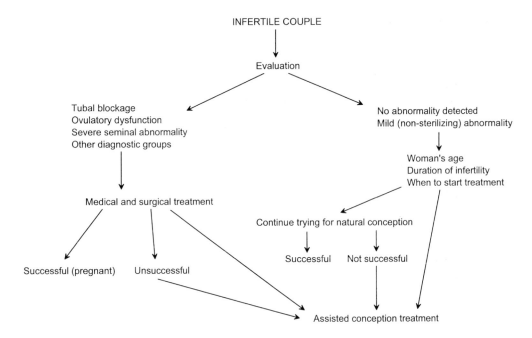

Figure 6.8. Decision-making in infertility management.

ample time to consider their options and embark on timely informed management pathways. Finally, early investigation of infertile couples should not lead to an unnecessarily high level of intervention. However, by identifying those that need immediate treatment (Figure 6.8) other couples will be in a better position to decide for themselves what their options are, having taken their individual characteristics into consideration.

BIBLIOGRAPHY

Bradshaw, K. D., Chantilis, S. J. & Carr, B. R. (1998). Diagnostic evaluation and treatment algorithms for the infertile couple. In *Textbook of Reproductive Medicine*, ed. B. R. Carr & R. E. Blackwell, 2nd edn, pp. 533–47. Stamford: Appleton & Lange.

McConnell, J. D. (1998). Diagnosis and treatment of male infertility. In *Textbook of Reproductive Medicine*, ed. B. R. Carr & R. E. Blackwell, 2nd edn, pp. 549–64. Stamford: Appleton & Lange.

Meniru, G. I., Brinsden, P. R. & Craft, I. L. (Eds) (1997). *A Handbook of Intrauterine Insemination*. Cambridge: Cambridge University Press.

Rebar, R. W. (1998). Assessment of the female patient. In *Textbook of Reproductive Medicine*, ed. B. R. Carr & R. E. Blackwell, 2nd edn, pp. 271–87. Stamford: Appleton & Lange.

Rowe, P. J., Comhaire, F. H., Hargreave, T. B. & Mellows, H. J. (1993). *WHO Manual for the Standardized Investigation and Diagnosis of the Infertile Couple.* Cambridge: Cambridge University Press.

Rowe, P. J., Comhaire, F. H., Hargreave, T. B. & Mahmoud, A. M. A. (2000). *WHO Manual for the Standardized Investigation, Diagnosis and Management of the Infertile Male.* Cambridge: Cambridge University Press.

Speroff, L., Glass, R. H. & Kase, N. G. (1999). Female infertility. In *Clinical Gynecologic Endocrinology and Infertility*, 6th edn, pp. 1013–42. Baltimore: Lippincott Williams & Wilkins.

Speroff, L., Glass, R. H. & Kase, N. G. (1999). Male infertility. In *Clinical Gynecologic Endocrinology and Infertility*, 6th edn, pp. 1075–96. Baltimore: Lippincott Williams & Wilkins.

World Health Organization (1992). *WHO Laboratory Manual for the Examination of Human Semen and Sperm–Cervical Mucus Interaction*, 3rd edn. Cambridge: Cambridge University Press.

World Health Organization (1999). *WHO Laboratory Manual for the Examination of Human Semen and Sperm–Cervical Mucus Interaction*, 4th edn. Cambridge: Cambridge University Press.

7

Medical and surgical treatment of infertility

Introduction

An understanding of presently available treatment options greatly simplifies the management of infertile couples. It is then easier to identify couples who will benefit from a particular type of treatment and those who will not. The basic infertility investigations have already been described and will identify most of the patients with any of the major causes of infertility. It is prudent to complete these investigations before offering treatment to any of the partners. There is always a temptation to postpone certain investigations, like laparoscopy and dye test and even hysterosalpingography, pending the outcome of some treatments such as induction of ovulation with clomiphene citrate for indicated or empirical reasons. Many would defend this practice on the basis of cost savings, and convenience for the patient but how would they defend a situation in which a woman has ovulation induction for several months only to discover that both her tubes are blocked? Furthermore, the current uncertainty regarding the relationship of ovulation induction and the later development of ovarian and female genital tract cancers should discourage unindicated use of ovulation induction agents.

Infertile couples have traditionally been inundated with remedies, most of which are of unproven benefit to their condition. The end result of the application of useless treatment modalities is that it prolongs the infertile state and as the woman gets older it becomes more difficult for usually efficacious techniques to succeed if and when they are eventually used. Worse still, inappropriate surgical intervention can worsen the infertile state by causing pelvic adhesions that involve the ovaries and fallopian tubes.

The treatment of infertility can be by means of medications, surgery and/or assisted conception methods. This chapter will deal with the first two methods while the rest of this book will deal with various aspects of assisted conception treatment. Most of the infertility problems that will be considered in the present chapter have already been discussed in relation to the causation and investigation of infertility in Chapters 4, 5 and 6.

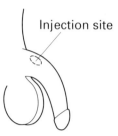

Injection site

Figure 7.1   Site of injection of agents such as papaverine, phentolamine and prostaglandin E$_1$ into the penis. The injection needs to be made into the corpus cavernosum.

Treatment of the male partner

Impotence

The treatment of impotence depends on the identified cause. A large proportion of cases will have a psychological basis, resulting from the interaction between the man's current problems and his past experiences. This will be further complicated by the stress of infertility and 'mechanization' of sex that invariably follows masturbation on demand at the infertility clinic and attempts at timing intercourse for the fertile period of the woman's cycle. Such men can still have erections during sleep. They have to be evaluated first of all by a psychologist with special interests in sexual dysfunction who will help to identify the origins of the man's problem. The couple will then be helped to gradually regain a relaxed and spontaneous approach towards sexual intercourse. During the initial part of sex therapy they are not allowed to have penetrative sexual intercourse; it is allowed only later, when the man has regained the ability to have a sustained erection without any feeling of anxiety or pressure to perform adequately.

Some cases of impotence will be caused by hormone-related problems such as hypogonadotrophic hypogonadism and hyperprolactinaemia. Treatment in such patients consists of replacing the missing hormone through injections or administering bromocriptine tablets if hyperprolactinaemia is the cause. Other causes of impotence such as diabetes, spinal cord injury and multiple sclerosis may not be reversible but affected patients can achieve erections by injecting agents like papaverine, phentolamine and prostaglandin E$_1$ into the penis (Figure 7.1). Vacuum and other erection devices can also be used but the latter may incorporate a rubber band that constricts the base of the penis and prevents normal ejaculation. This makes them unsuitable for achieving intravaginal ejaculation. Devices can be implanted in the penis to confer some rigidity that will allow its insertion into the vagina. Operations can also be performed on the penis to restore its normal blood supply if a defective blood supply is shown to be the problem. Electroejaculation will be described in the following sections. While this procedure does not cure impotence it will lead to the production of semen for use in assisted conception treatment.

Of great interest internationally has been the recent clinical availability of viagra tablets (Sildenafil citrate, Pfizer Ltd) for use in the treatment of impotence and other problems which together constitute erectile dysfunction. Viagra is a potent inhibitor of the enzyme, phosphodiesterase type 5 (PDE5), that metabolizes cyclic guanosine monophosphate (cGMP). cGMP is involved in the erection mechanism of the penis; it induces relaxation of the corpus carvenosal smooth muscle thereby leading to engorgement of the penis and erection. When PDE5 is inhibited by viagra, the level of cGMP increases in the penis resulting in a natural erectile response to sexual stimulation. Preliminary data has been highly laudatory of the efficacy of viagra with significant improvement being documented in the ability of patients to achieve and maintain erections. Viagra is available in 25 mg, 50 mg and 100 mg tablets and is taken orally one hour before sexual intercourse. Just ingesting the drug will not lead to an erection; there needs to be sexual stimulation. More clinical experience is accruing regarding the type of patients who will benefit from the use of this drug. For the time being satisfactory responses have been noted in patients with psychogenic impotence as well as those whose impotence is due to diabetes, bilateral nerve sparing radical prostatectomy (Zippe et al., 1998), spinal cord injury occurring between T6 and L5 (Derry et al., 1998) and some other organic causes of impotence. Adverse effects include headache, flushing, dyspepsia, rhinitis and abnormal colour vision. Priapism is an uncommon problem (Viera et al., 1999). Viagra can cause hypotension; its ingestion by a patient who is also on organic nitrates (for example nitroglycerin) or uses amyl nitrite for recreational purposes, may lead to a catastrophic fall in the blood pressure. The use of viagra is contraindicated in these patients. Individuals with known or suspected heart disease, hypotension, hypovolaemia, or other risk factors such as multi-drug antihypertensive therapy, should have a full clinical review and cardiac testing before a decision is made on who can have the drug. Other patients with known chronic ailments should have a full clinical review before being prescribed viagra. Similar assessments should be carried out on any patient who is on drugs that are metabolized by or inhibit cytochrome P450 enzyme 3A4 before deciding on whether to prescribe viagra (Viera et al., 1999).

Retrograde ejaculation

If retrograde ejaculation is linked to any medication that the patient is taking, stopping its continued use may result in a return to normal functioning. In cases where no cause is found or the patient has problems such as diabetes, a trial of treatment with pseudoephedrine and imipramine tablets may be successful. Some patients have been successfully treated by having them ejaculate with full bladders (Crich &

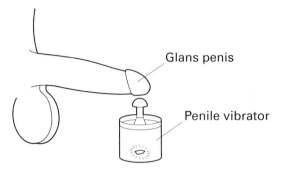

Glans penis

Penile vibrator

Figure 7.2   A penile vibrator being applied to the glans penis.

Jequier, 1978). The rationale for this treatment is that continence of urine with a full bladder involves closure of the bladder sphincters; this implies that the backward flow of semen into the bladder at the time of ejaculation will be prevented by these sphincters. In patients where other treatments have failed, sodium bicarbonate is dissolved in water and drunk some hours beforehand. This makes the urine alkaline and less toxic to sperm. The man then empties the bladder before having intercourse or masturbating. Following orgasm he urinates into a clean sterile plastic container. This is immediately taken to the laboratory for the extraction of spermatozoa. These will either be used immediately for assisted conception treatment or frozen for later use. If retrograde ejaculation is associated with impotence or a lack of ejaculation, a catheter is used to empty the bladder before and after ejaculation or emission following vibratory or electrical stimulation. Gamete culture medium, containing antibiotics, is used to rinse the bladder. A small amount of the fresh culture medium is then left in the bladder. Following ejaculation the catheter is passed into the bladder again and used to remove the fluid which should contain spermatozoa.

Anejaculation

Ejaculatory failure is also known as anejaculation. Its spectrum of causes mirrors that of impotence. Treatment can be with the use of medications such as pseudoephedrine and imipramine. Other groups of patients may require the use of stimulatory methods to achieve emission. The two popular stimulatory methods are penile vibratory stimulation and rectal electrostimulation. In the first method, a penile vibrator is applied to the glans penis (Figure 7.2) while in the second method a probe is carefully passed into the rectum, placed against the site of the seminal vesicles and intermittent electrical currents applied (Figure 7.3). The electrical current stimulates the muscles in the seminal vesicles as well as those in the prostate, vas deferens and epididymis to contract and expel semen into the urethra.

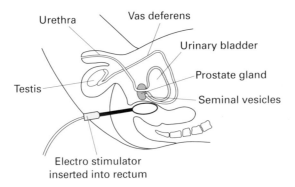

Urethra

Vas deferens

Urinary bladder

Prostate gland

Testis

Seminal vesicles

Electro stimulator
inserted into rectum

Figure 7.3   Application of a rectal electrostimulator to induce emission of semen.

Urine is alkalinized beforehand and the bladder rinsed with culture medium as described above. Following stimulation and emission the semen is milked out of the urethra and collected in a sterile plastic container. The bladder is then catheterized to remove the fluid previously left there, which may now contain spermatozoa.

These methods can cause complications which should be described to the patient carefully before he gives his consent for the procedure. The main complication, which is known as autonomic hyperreflexia, is characterized by a rapidly rising blood pressure following orgasm. This can be prevented by prior administration of drugs such as nifedipine. Other problems include perforation of the rectum with the probe, bleeding from the rectum after electrostimulation and burns to the walls of the rectum due to the probe getting very hot during use. Some patients either have urinary retention or develop urinary tract infection. Alternatives to these procedures include aspiration of spermatozoa directly from the epididymis, vas deferens or testis. The surgical sperm retrieval methods are described in Chapter 10.

Antisperm antibodies in the man

The medical treatment of infertility resulting from the production of antisperm antibodies by the man has proved disappointing. Attempts have been made to administer steroids to the man with the hope that this will suppress his immunity to the extent that he stops producing antisperm antibodies. Various researchers have published conflicting results; some say that this form of treatment works while a large majority have not found a higher pregnancy rate from steroid treatment. Furthermore, the required long-term treatment with high doses of steroids has deleterious effects on the body and could cause hypertension, excessive salt and water retention, diabetes, osteoporosis (bone loss), bone fractures, mental disturbances, peptic ulcers, Cushing's syndrome, poor immunity to infections, muscle wasting and so many other problems. The present consensus of opinion is that assisted conception treatment is a better option for this group of patients if infertility is prolonged. It has to be stated again that antisperm antibodies are a relative and not an absolute cause of infertility. Many couples with this problem are still able to establish pregnancies naturally within a reasonable length of time. It is only in those who fail to do so that assisted conception treatment may be indicated.

Hypogonadotrophic hypogonadism

Patients with this problem have to be investigated to exclude causes that require treatment such as brain tumours. It is only after this evaluation that hormone replacement therapy can be used in either of two broad approaches. The patient can be administered gonadotrophin releasing hormone (GnRH) using a continuous infusion pump with the needle being placed subcutaneously (under the skin and in the fat layer). The pump is programmed to deliver small doses of the drug at set intervals just as occurs in the natural state. Alternatively, human chorionic gonadotrophin (hCG) and/or human menopausal gonadotrophin (hMG) can be administered two to three times a week. Both approaches will need prolonged use to stimulate adequate production of spermatozoa and up to two years may be required for this to happen in some cases.

Hyperprolactinaemia

The treatment of hyperprolactinaemia will be considered in greater detail in relation to the female. In summary, the clinical history will identify male patients who are currently on medications that are recognized causes of hyperprolactinaemia. Brain scans are required to diagnose or exclude pituitary tumours. Following this bromocriptine tablets or suitable alternatives are administered to decrease production of prolactin. Other treatment modalities include surgery and radiotherapy but these will only be required in a very select group of patients.

Accessory gland infection

Acute infection of any of the male accessory sex glands is usually characterized by fever, a feeling of malaise, pain in the location of the particular gland and other symptoms depending on which gland is affected. Diagnosis is aided by microbiological culture of urine specimens and urethral discharge. Treatment is by means of antibiotics.

In some men no obvious symptoms are present yet semen samples contain more white blood cells than is normal. Culture of semen may not reveal any micro-organism. Opinion is divided as to whether to give antibiotics to such men. This is because antibiotic treatment may not lead to a reduction of the high concentration

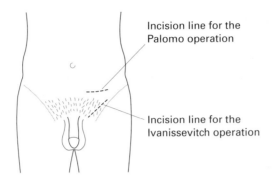

Incision line for the
Palomo operation

Incision line for the
Ivanissevitch operation

Figure 7.4 Two approaches for varicocoelectomy. In the Ivanissevitch operation an incision is made in the mid-portion of the inguinal canal while in the Palomo operation the incision is made at a higher level (level of the iliac crest).

of white blood cells. Moreover antibiotics themselves are increasingly being shown to depress the production of spermatozoa.

Varicocoele

The surgical treatment of varicocoele is aimed at blocking the internal spermatic vein on the affected side. This commonly involves making an incision in the lower aspect of the abdominal wall near the pubis or just above the groin (Figure 7.4). The vein is identified, tied up and cut. Another approach is the use of X-ray techniques such as fluoroscopy to guide a catheter to the affected internal spermatic vein where chemical agents, spring coils or balloons are released to cause blockage of the vein. Others use the laparoscope to tie and cut the internal spermatic vein. Complications after these procedures include wound infection, recurrence of the varicocoele, hydrocoele formation (fluid collection around the testes), infection of the epididymis and rarely, atrophy of the testes.

The treatment of varicocoele is controversial because there is disagreement regarding the relationship of varicocoele to infertility. Varicocoeles can be found in men who have had no problems having children but the incidence amongst male partners in infertile couples is higher. The relationship may not be straightforward and requires further study to clarify issues. There is certainly a subgroup of men with abnormal semen parameters who have no other apparent cause for the problem except for the existence of a varicocoele. The testis on the affected side is usually smaller in size. Such men are likely to benefit from surgical treatment of the varicocoele. The men will show improvements in their semen parameters after the operation and it may take up to two years for the full impact of the operation to be realized in some cases. The finding of a varicocoele does not exempt the female partner from being evaluated, since there may be co-existing female factor problems.

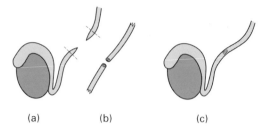

(a)   (b)   (c)

Figure 7.5   Vasovasostomy: (a) excision of the blocked portion(s) of the vas deferens; (b) cut ends of the vas deferens; and, (c) rejoining of the healthy portions of the vas deferens using fine sutures.

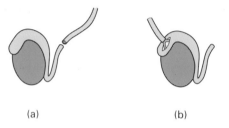

(a)   (b)

Figure 7.6   Vasoepididymostomy: (a) the vas deferens is freed by cutting it near to its point of origin; followed by, (b) attachment of the cut end to a dilated epididymal tubule.

Obstructive azoospermia

Blockage of the male genital tract as a result of vasectomy or as a complication of other operations such as hernia repair and hydrocoelectomy can at times be treated successfully by surgery. In the procedure known as vasovasostomy, the affected part of the vas deferens is excised and the normal portions rejoined using fine sutures (Figure 7.5). In vasoepididymostomy a blocked part of the epididymis is bypassed by joining the cut end of the vas deferens to an epididymal tubule in which motile spermatozoa have been identified after making a tiny incision on the wall of the tubule (Figure 7.6). Obstruction of the ejaculatory duct can often be relieved by an incision made with the aid of an operating cystoscope that is passed into the urethra (Figure 7.7). These and similar operations have allowed men with obstructive azoospermia to have children naturally. There are however a large group of men in whom the operation fails or is not possible due to the nature of the blockage. The latter group include men with congenital absence of both vasa deferentia. Previously these men could not have children of their own but latest assisted conception techniques have now made genetic parenthood possible for them by surgical sperm retrieval. These techniques will be described in later chapters.

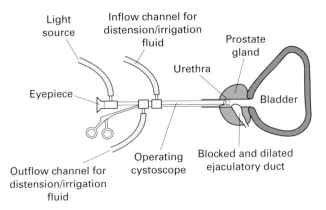

Figure 7.7   An operating cystoscope is introduced into the urethra for use in making an incision into a blocked ejaculatory duct.

In patients with irremediable obstructive azoospermia attempts have been made to implant a device which is connected to a patent part of the epididymis. This device is called an alloplastic spermatocoele and it acts as a reservoir for collecting spermatozoa that are produced by the testis to which it is connected. The intention is for the spermatocoele to be aspirated at intervals and the recovered spermatozoa used for assisted conception treatment. Alloplastic spermatocoeles have not been very successful for long-term management of these patients. This is because they tend to become blocked within a very short time of insertion. In fact spermatocoeles should be aspirated within three to five days of insertion because they start to become occluded after about one week.

A large proportion of males with long-standing obstructive azoospermia develop antisperm antibodies. Even in cases in which patency of the vas deferens is restored with any of the above treatments and spermatozoa reappear in the ejaculate, the presence of antisperm antibodies may still depress fertility and prevent natural conception; such couples will eventually require assisted conception treatment.

Azoospermia not due to obstruction

When non-appearance of spermatozoa in the ejaculate is not due to blockage at any point along the male genital tract the patient is said to have non-obstructive or secretory azoospermia. Most cases will be due to a failure of the testes to produce spermatozoa because of an intrinsic problem with the testes (primary testicular failure) but cases of hypogonadotrophic hypogonadism (secondary testicular failure) have to be excluded by relevant laboratory tests. In the former case the level of follicle stimulating hormone (FSH) and luteinizing hormone (LH) will be high, while in the latter case these hormones are non-detectable in blood. There is no medical therapy that is currently available for patients with primary testicular failure and in past years parentage for such men could only be achieved through the use of donor sperm insemination of his partner or adoption. However, it has been found recently that a few spermatozoa can be recovered from the testes of some of these men. This often involves prolonged dissection and careful examination of testicular tissue removed surgically from the man's testes. It has been possible for these few spermatozoa to be used for assisted conception treatment and result in pregnancy.

Other considerations

Men with decreased semen parameters of undiagnosed origin have been traditionally asked to wear loose boxer shorts and have intermittent cold baths to help reduce the temperature of the testes. This advice is based on the belief that this will increase production of spermatozoa. However, there is presently no strong evidence to show that these measures improve the semen quality. Men in infertile relationships, especially those with unexplained subnormal semen parameters, should avoid soaking in hot tubs. Tobacco smoking, use of marijuana and excessive alcohol intake depress production of spermatozoa. While it is true that some heavy smokers and alcoholics father children, the effect of these and other factors on the genesis of infertility problems is not easy to predict and may depend more on individual susceptibility. Some of the deleterious effects may be time dependent; it may take some years for the production of spermatozoa to be depressed to such an extent that infertility arises. Furthermore, those who already have borderline semen parameters may more readily become infertile when compared to those with much better initial semen parameters. It is strongly advised, therefore, that these habits should be stopped. There is an ever expanding list of debilitating and life threatening diseases also associated with their use. Cessation of the use of anabolic steroids or other culpable medications may lead to an improvement of the semen quality while the effect of stopping certain medications, such as anticancer drugs, may take a longer time to manifest. Some men have been empirically administered various vitamins (especially vitamins C and E), minerals (e.g. zinc), hormone injections, antibiotics and other medications. There is currently no unanimity regarding their efficacy. Vitamins C and E may be marginally effective in some men; it certainly does no harm if patients take these vitamins in reasonable quantities. However, some of the other preparations may worsen the state of infertility and should be avoided – for example, antibiotics, which are increasingly being shown to depress production of spermatozoa.

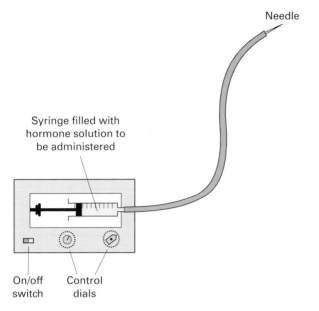

Figure 7.8   Diagram showing key components of the syringe pump set-up used for the pulsatile administration of gonadotrophin releasing hormone.

Treatment of the female partner

Exercise and weight loss induced ovulatory dysfunction

Ovulatory problems resulting from underweight or strenuous exercise are brought about by a decrease in the secretion of GnRH by the hypothalamus. Increasing food intake and decreasing the intensity of exercise will lead to weight gain and an increase in the proportion of body fat and hence a restoration of normal secretory patterns of GnRH by the hypothalamus.

Hypogonadotrophic hypogonadism

The most common method used in managing this problem, which is also highly effective, is by the pulsatile administration of GnRH using a syringe pump (Figure 7.8) (Tan & Jacobs, 1991; Balen & Jacobs, 1997). This technique mimics the natural situation since this same hormone is not secreted continuously by the hypothalamus but in pulses (intermittently) every 71–94 minutes in the follicular phase and every 103–216 minutes in the luteal phase of the menstrual cycle. The syringe pump is battery driven and can be programmed to deliver different volumes of fluid at various intervals. It is worn on a belt tied around the waist and delivers the drug to the body through a tubing that ends in a needle. This needle is normally pushed through the skin and into the underlying fat layer of the arm. The needle can also be inserted into a vein but this makes the treatment more invasive and exposes the patient to a greater risk of developing blood-borne infection (bacteraemia). Moreover, the patient can learn to insert the needle into the fat layer of the skin by herself. Siting the needle in a vein requires that the patient goes to the hospital for the nurse or doctor to do this every few days.

The syringe containing the GnRH solution is loaded onto the syringe pump. Different rates of administration of GnRH have been used by various workers and they lie within the range of 1–20 mg/pulse at 90–120 minute intervals. The pulsatile administration of GnRH to the patient stimulates secretion of FSH and LH by the pituitary gland. These gonadotrophins then act on the ovaries to stimulate follicular development as well as the secretion of oestrogen in the follicular phase, and both oestrogen and progesterone in the luteal phase. The response to treatment is monitored mainly with ultrasound scanning. The first scan is performed before starting the GnRH administration. Another scan is then carried out on Day 10, and subsequently every other day until ovulation occurs. These scans track the number of developing follicles and their diameter. Some authorities recommend carrying out a Day 21 progesterone assay to confirm ovulation in that first cycle; if ovulation is documented each subsequent treatment cycle is monitored with fewer ultrasound scans and a Day 21 progesterone assay. Ovulation is triggered with the administration of hCG injection when the follicle reaches a diameter of 18 mm or above. Sexual intercourse is timed to occur on the day hCG is administered, the day after and, if possible, also the next day. The GnRH infusion is continued (with the frequency of administration decreased to about once every four hours) during the luteal phase to support the development and function of the corpus luteum. Alternatively, hCG is administered together with GnRH during the luteal phase.

The use of pulsatile GnRH administration is highly effective. Up to 90% of females with hypogonadotrophic hypogonadism ovulate. About 90% of those who ovulate become pregnant within the first six months of treatment. This is provided there is no male factor problem or any untreated female factor problem. Induction of ovulation can also be carried out with the administration of hMG. The technique will be described in the following section under polycystic ovary syndrome. About 90% of patients will ovulate on the hMG treatment regimen and the conception rate is about 85% during the first year of treatment. However, as will be seen in later sections and the chapters on assisted conception treatment, stimulation of follicular development and ovulation is associated with certain complications. These include ovarian hyperstimulation syndrome (OHSS), multiple pregnancies and possibly an increase in the incidence of miscarriage in those who become pregnant. If the correct procedure is followed, pulsatile GnRH administration usually leads to the ovulation of one oocyte, so the incidence of multiple pregnancy is low (5–8%), and not very dissimilar to that in the general population. The chance of developing OHSS is almost non-existent. Whether the incidence of miscarriage (29%) is higher than the background miscarriage rate in the general population is still debatable. Infection of the site of needle insertion is not common and is easily managed by removing the needle from that site and inserting a fresh needle at another site. When hMG is used for induction of ovulation instead of GnRH the multiple pregnancy rate is higher and the risk of having OHSS greater.

Polycystic ovary syndrome

More is being discovered about the disorders that make up the polycystic ovary syndrome (PCOS). What is emerging is a disease complex with numerous manifestations and affecting different organ systems in the body to varying extents. Even if such patients are not desirous of pregnancy they should still have regular medical check-ups because they have a higher tendency towards developing glucose intolerance or non-insulin dependent diabetes mellitus later in life. They also run the risk of developing hypertension, dyslipidaemia, atherosclerotic heart disease and myocardial infarction. Many of these females have long intervals between periods (oligomenorrhoea) or no menstrual periods at all (amenorrhoea). Their endometrium is exposed to the action of oestrogen for long periods of time and this exposes them to a higher risk of developing endometrial hyperplasia, and cancer of the endometrium, again in later life. Normally, ovulation is associated with the production of progesterone which then acts on the endometrium to modify the actions of oestrogen. The shedding of the top layers of the endometrium during menstrual periods each month follows the fall in the level of the two hormones in the late luteal phase. Therefore even though fertility may not be desired in some cases of PCOS it must be ensured that the patients have at least three to four normal menstrual periods in a year. If need be, they are administered progesterone, in the form of tablets, for 14 days in the luteal phase or whenever the periods are long overdue and a sensitive pregnancy test shows they are not pregnant. This induces an artificial menstrual period, called withdrawal bleeding, which is adequate for the purpose of reducing the risk of endometrial cancer in later life. Another aspect of the management of PCOS relates to the woman's weight. About 50% of PCOS patients are obese. While obesity may not necessarily cause PCOS it certainly worsens the manifestations of the disorder and weight loss improves the condition. Some patients may even start having normal menstrual periods when they lose weight. Even if normal ovulatory periods do not return, ovulation induction is easier to carry out when the weight returns to normal levels. The methods of ovulation induction usually employed in patients with PCOS include the administration of clomiphene citrate or tamoxifen tablets, pulsatile GnRH administration, gonadotrophin injections and ovarian diathermy. The use of insulin sensitizing agents such as metformin is now being investigated as a means of treating hyper-insulinaemia that is found in many of these patients.

Clomiphene citrate

Clomiphene citrate (CC) is a very popular agent for the induction of ovulation and has been in use for more than 35 years. It has a structure that shares key similarities with that of oestrogen. This enables CC to bind with receptors in the hypothalamus and pituitary and prevent oestrogen from binding with those same receptors. Because of this, the hypothalamus does not receive feedback information on the actual level of oestrogen in the body. The absence of such signals will be interpreted by the hypothalamus to mean that there is no oestrogen in the body. This leads to increased output of GnRH by the hypothalamus and consequently FSH and LH by the pituitary. The net result of these changes will be the production of one or more oocytes by the ovary. Treatment with CC is commenced at 50 mg daily for five days in each menstrual cycle. Many practitioners now prescribe this tablet to be taken on Days 2, 3, 4, 5 and 6 of the cycle. Others may commence the administration on either Day 3, 4 or 5. The patient's response to the treatment can be monitored with a combination of ultrasound scans and Day 21 progesterone assays. There is a chance that these women will initiate a spontaneous surge of LH secretion towards mid-cycle. This surge can usually be detected with urinary test kits, as the hormone also appears in urine. The use of these LH test kits will be described in greater detail in Chapter 8; urinary LH detection aids the timing of intercourse and Day 21 progesterone assay is used to confirm ovulation. It is quite important to use these monitoring techniques in the first two cycles of treatment with CC. This is to document the efficacy of the dose of CC that is being used. In subsequent cycles the couple can time intercourse using the calendar method and feedback from the first two cycles that were monitored more closely. Alternatively, the woman can check for the appearance of the pre-ovulatory mucus and time sexual intercourse appropriately. If the woman does not have a period after Day 35, a pregnancy test is carried out. If negative, she is administered a progestogen such as medroxyprogesterone acetate to induce a withdrawal bleed. Administration of CC is then started on Day 2 of the new cycle.

The dose of CC is increased to 100 mg in the next cycle of treatment if the woman does not ovulate on the 50 mg daily dose. If she still does not ovulate on the 100 mg dose she is kept on that dose for the next two cycles of treatment before being classified as being unresponsive to treatment with CC. Some practitioners will raise the dose up to 250 mg daily but this does not seem to confer any advantage. Rather some of the undesirable effects of CC, such as thickening of the cervical mucus to the extent that it is impenetrable by spermatozoa, will become manifest at these

Table 7.1. Side-effects of clomiphene citrate

Visual disturbances
Ovarian hyperstimulation
Hot flushes
Abdominal discomfort
Nausea
Vomiting
Depression
Insomnia
Breast tenderness
Weight gain
Rashes
Dizziness
Hair loss

Source: British National Formulary (1999).

high doses. If the patient ovulates on the 50–100 mg daily dose range she is maintained on the drug regimen for a total of six cycles of treatment. If she does not become pregnant the treatment will have to be reassessed and possibly changed to one of the assisted conception treatments. A case can be made for maintaining CC treatment for a total of 9–12 months in highly selected patients.

Treatment with CC is generally effective and up to 80% of females with PCOS will ovulate on the 50–100 mg daily dose regimen. About 33% of patients will become pregnant after five cycles of treatment. The multiple pregnancy rate is 5% and OHSS is uncommon. Females with PCOS have a higher incidence of miscarriage when they become pregnant. This is irrespective of the drug that was used in stimulating ovulation. This heightened risk of miscarriage is thought to be related to the high LH concentration that these patients tend to have which may exert deleterious effects on the oocyte during its development within the ovarian follicle.

CC has some side-effects associated with its use and they are listed in Table 7.1. Most of the problems are uncommon and do not necessarily mean cessation of therapy except for visual disturbances when treatment with CC should be stopped immediately. CC should not be given to females who have liver disease, ovarian cysts, endometrial cancer or abnormal uterine bleeding. It should also not be administered to women who are already pregnant. Tamoxifen is another drug which is similar to CC and can be administered to women with PCOS to induce ovulation. The dose is 20–40 mg taken on Days 2, 3, 4, 5 and 6 just like CC. Tamoxifen and CC will not be effective in patients with hypogonadotrophic hypogonadism.

GnRH

Although GnRH can be administered to females with PCOS there are some differences in technique from that used for females with hypogonadotrophic hypogonadism. The pulsatile administration of GnRH with an infusion pump is
commenced with the onset of menstrual periods or withdrawal bleeding. The
response to ovarian stimulation is monitored with ultrasound scanning and
urinary LH detection. When the LH surge is detected it means that the patient is
likely to ovulate within 24–36 hours. She should have sexual intercourse on the day
the LH surge is detected and the following day to ensure the presence of live motile
spermatozoa in the female genital tract by the time the ovulated oocyte enters the
fallopian tube or shortly thereafter. At times the LH surge that occurs in cycles in
which drugs are administered to stimulate the ovaries, is suboptimal and the
hormone level is inadequate for the final maturation and ovulation of the oocyte.
This is why some practitioners will administer hCG immediately the LH surge is
detected to ensure the completion of events started by LH. In cases where the LH
surge is not detected by the time the developing follicle reaches a diameter of
18 mm or above, hCG injection can be given to trigger off ovulation. Ovulation
induction with pulsatile GnRH is not as successful in PCOS patients as it is in
females who have hypogonadotrophic hypogonadism. In one study, ovulation was
successfully induced in 41.7% of the treatment cycles and conception occurred in
13% of the patients.

Gonadotrophins

Gonodotrophins may be administered to PCOS patients either as first line treatment or, more commonly, as a second option for those who fail to ovulate on CC.
For a long time the gonadotrophin preparations that were available for use in infertility treatments were extracted from the urine of menopausal women. As was noted
in Chapters 5 and 6, the pituitary gland secretes large amounts of FSH and LH when
the ovaries start failing and this high level of production is maintained for many
years after the menopause. The extracted hormones are packaged in ampoules containing FSH and LH in a 1:1 ratio. These preparations were called human menopausal gonadotrophins or hMG. The amount of each hormone in an ampoule of
hMG is usually 75 international units (IU) (i.e. LH = 75 IU; FSH = 75 IU).

Further experience with ovulation induction suggested that women with PCOS
especially, who already have high levels of LH, might have deleterious effects from
additional exogenous LH. This led to the development of preparations in which
most of the LH had been removed. These were called 'pure' FSH and contained 75
IU of the hormone in each ampoule. It has since been found that 'pure' FSH preparations can also be administered to patients who do not have PCOS. This is
because the ovaries do not need the relatively large amounts of LH contained in

hMG injections to produce sufficient numbers of oocytes and concentrations of oestrogen. However, these injections cannot be given to women with hypogonadotrophic hypogonadism because they need at least some LH to ovulate normally.

The collection of urine for the production of urinary gonadotrophin injections has not been the most aesthetically appealing activity. Coupled with other problems, such as shortage of menopausal urine! and the risk of viral transmission, there was a stimulus for the development of more suitable means of producing gonadotrophins for human use. Production of FSH injections through genetic engineering was eventually developed and these are now available for use. Commercial production of genetically engineered LH is near completion.

Induction of ovulation with gonadotrophins in females with PCOS and others is still far from a perfect science. This is because each female responds differently to the same dose of gonadotrophin and identification of the ideal dosage is by trial and error. It is important to achieve a good level of control over the effective dosage of gonadotrophins because induction of ovulation aims at the production of one oocyte in each cycle of treatment similar to the natural situation. When this number is exceeded the multiple pregnancy rate escalates. Up to a quarter of women who get pregnant following induction of ovulation with gonadotrophins have multiple pregnancies. The incidence of OHSS is also higher.

The regimen for induction of ovulation in both PCOS patients and other patients consists of the administration of hMG and/or FSH injections from Day 2 of the menstrual cycle or withdrawal bleeding. One ampoule (i.e. 75 IU) is administered daily or two ampoules (150 IU) injected every other day. The most important monitoring tool is the ultrasound scan. Some practitioners also use hormone assays while many others do not feel there is any practical reason for carrying out hormone assays except for research and for patients with special problems. It is important to watch out for the LH surge and urine LH testing should be commenced from about Day 9. Sexual intercourse should be timed to take place on the day the LH surge is detected and on the following day. The LH surge can be supported with an injection of hCG. This same injection is also administered if the surge is not detected by the time a follicle reaches the diameter of 18 mm or above. Sexual intercourse should take place on the day of hCG injection and the day afterwards. Research has shown that PCOS patients who are treated with gonadotrophins because of their lack of response to CC have a 75% chance of ovulating. Another study showed that 62% of the women conceived in the six months of treatment while 73% did so by the twelfth month. The multiple pregnancy rate following treatment with gonadotrophins is about 20%. The risk of OHSS is more real with gonadotrophin administration and up to 15% of women will have some degree of the problem. However, it is only about 1% who will have the severe variety necessitating hospital admission and intensive care. The use of gonadotrophins is often left to the experienced reproductive specialist because of its risks and unpredictability.

Ovarian diathermy

Prior to the discovery of the drugs that are used nowadays for induction of ovulation the only effective means of inducing ovulation in females with PCOS was to remove a piece of tissue from the ovary. The operation was called wedge resection of the ovary. It was unclear why this operation worked but many women ovulated after the operation and some became pregnant. A major problem with this operation was that there was a tendency for adhesions to form between the ovary and the other pelvic organs such as the fallopian tubes, thereby jeopardising the woman's fertility further. This operation was largely discontinued following the advent of reliable drugs for ovarian stimulation.

There has been a recent reawakening of interest in the use of surgical means to induce ovulation in women with PCOS. This is because of the fact that some women will not respond to CC treatment while others over-respond to hMG/FSH injections. Furthermore, there have been increasing reports of a possible association between ovarian cancer and the use of drugs for the induction of ovulation. It is hoped that these problems will be avoided if the patient is made to ovulate spontaneously following surgical treatment. For the time being, the main indication for ovarian diathermy is a lack of response, by a patient with PCOS, to the use of CC. Holes are drilled in one or both ovaries, under laparoscopic guidance, using diathermy (metal probes that generate high temperatures when an electrical current is passed through them) or laser. Ovulation rates following this procedure is in the region of 80% and it seems to decrease the tonically high levels of LH commonly found in women with PCOS (Balen & Jacobs, 1997). There is a risk of peri-ovarian adhesion formation following this procedure but the incidence seems to be low (10–20%).

Hyperprolactinaemia

The management of hyperprolactinaemia depends to some extent on the primary cause of the problem, if it can be detected, and associated manifestations such as amenorrhoea and infertility. Discontinuation of an offending drug (see Chapter 5) such as metoclopramide or substitution with another drug that does not cause hyperprolactinaemia, may be all that is needed to reduce the prolactin level to normal. In some situations a suitable alternative may not be found, in which case use of the offending drug is continued with regular checks of the blood concentration of prolactin; hormone replacement therapy for oestrogen deficiency is performed using oral contraceptives. Treatment of any causative disorder such as hypothyroidism and brain infections could also lead to restoration of normal prolactin levels.

Table 7.2. Side-effects of bromocriptine

Normal doses of bromocriptine	High doses of bromocriptine
Nausea and vomiting	Confusion
Constipation	Psychomotor excitation
Headache	Hallucinations
Dizziness	Dyskinesia
Postural hypotension	Dry mouth
Drowsiness	Leg cramps
Vasospasm of fingers and toes (especially in patients with Raynaud's syndrome)	Pleural effusion (accumulation of fluid in the chest but outside the lungs)
	Retroperitoneal fibrosis

Source: British National Formulary (1999).

Medical treatment

For other patients, medical treatment is the first option while surgery and radiation treatment are reserved for a small proportion of unresponsive patients. Bromocriptine is the mainstay of drug treatment of hyperprolactinaemia in the absence of a medically correctable cause as noted above. It belongs to the group of drugs called dopamine agonists and has been in clinical use for more than 20 years. The dose of the drug is 2.5 mg up to three times daily but smaller doses are usually administered initially to avoid precipitation of side-effects. Different practitioners vary in the way they start administration of the drug but the following regimen is popular. Bromocriptine is administered with meals at night using a dose of 1.25 mg every night for three days. Provided no side-effects manifest (Table 7.2), the dose is increased to 2.5 mg taken once at night for one week. After this time 2.5 mg is administered at night and once during the day time, again with meals. The dose is then increased, after about a week, to 2.5 mg administered three times daily. The dose can be increased to a maximum total daily dose of 30 mg.

Some workers have reported on intravaginal administration of bromocriptine tablets as an alternative in females who do not tolerate its oral administration (Vermesh et al., 1988; Ginsburg et al., 1992). A single 2.5 mg tablet is inserted high up in the vagina at night just before going to bed. There is adequate absorption of the drug into the blood circulation and blood levels are maintained for up to 24 hours. More importantly treatment with a single intravaginal 2.5 mg dose each day was found to reduce the prolactin level in 90% of patients normalizing the levels in 30% of cases. A monthly bromocriptine injection has been developed but has not yet been used in clinical practice (Balen & Jacobs, 1997; Mishell, 1997).

It may take about 6–10 weeks for the beneficial effects of bromocriptine to manifest in women who have hyperprolactinaemia that is not the result of pituitary tumours; the prolactin level drops, galactorrhoea resolves and the menstrual periods resume. Ovulation usually resumes in these women. Once a clinical response is noted the dose of the drug should be reduced, as most women will continue to respond adequately to a lower maintenance dose of bromocriptine. It may take up to 10–16 weeks for the effects of bromocriptine to be noted in women who have pituitary microadenoma. However, bromocriptine is effective in these and other women who have pituitary tumours as the cause of the hyperprolactinaemia and leads to shrinkage of the tumour in more than 90% of cases (Tan & Jacobs, 1991). Those tumours that do not shrink are most likely to be tumours that do not secrete prolactin but produce hyperprolactinaemia by compressing the hypothalamus thereby interrupting the control pathways through which the hypothalamus inhibits the production of prolactin by the pituitary gland.

Although bromocriptine seems to be safe in pregnancy it is usually recommended that administration of the drug is discontinued in women who become pregnant even if they have macroadenoma since there is no significant enlargement of these tumours during pregnancy. However, evidence of tumour growth is sought by regularly examining the patient's visual fields throughout pregnancy and performing a limited MRI (magnetic resonance imaging) scan whenever an abnormality is detected (Schlaff & Kletzky, 1998).

Cabergoline and quinagolide are two other medications that can be used in place of bromocriptine for treating hyperprolactinaemia. Their appeal mainly lies in the fact that they have fewer side-effects and may be tolerated more by patients who react to the use of bromocriptine. The administration of cabergoline can be restricted to once or twice a week while that of quinagolide mirrors that of bromocriptine.

Long-term treatment (one to two years) with bromocriptine is carried out in women who are not immediately desirous of having children. One of the advantages of this regimen is that it may provide a permanent cure for hyperprolactinaemia in 10–20% of females who have or do not have associated microadenomas. Even where a permanent cure is not achieved the blood concentration of prolactin does not return to the pre-treatment value in a significant proportion of patients. Long-term medical treatment is also advocated for patients with responsive macroadenomas and has been used for up to 12 years in some cases (Mishell, 1997).

Surgical treatment

Surgery (transphenoidal resection of tumour) is reserved for patients with macroadenomas that do not respond to medical treatment or non-functioning tumours. Another indication for surgery is when side-effects of drug treatment are intolerable but various drug manipulations should be tried before resorting to surgery.

This operation has a low mortality rate of less than 0.5%. However 10–40% of patients may have temporary diabetes insipidus. In this condition the patient passes large volumes of dilute urine because of an inability to reabsorb fluid in the kidneys. Most patients recover from this with only 2% having a persistent problem (Mishell, 1997). The operation can, in another 2% of cases, lead to damage of other parts of the pituitary leading to a condition called panhypopituitarism in which all the hormones normally produced by the pituitary gland have to be administered artificially to maintain normal body functions. The initial cure rate following surgery is quoted at between 65 and 85% for microadenomas and 20 and 40% for macroadenomas (Mishell, 1997) but a significant proportion of patients (20–80%) have a recurrence of the problem. This is one of the reasons why drug treatment should always be aimed for in women with hyperprolactinaemia.

Radiation treatment

Tumour irradiation can be achieved using either external beam therapy or by implanting radioisotopes (radiation emitting compounds) in the pituitary. The treatment has not been satisfactory because tissue destruction cannot be controlled precisely and parts of normal pituitary tissue may be destroyed. This could lead to diabetes insipidus and panhypopituitarism. Some patients have had visual problems following this treatment as a result of damage to the optic nerves (Mishel, 1997; Schlaff & Kletzky, 1998). Radiotherapy is usually reserved for patients in whom there is incomplete surgical removal of non-drug responsive tumour tissue.

Ovarian failure/resistant ovary syndrome

This is one area where practitioners need to be very humane in their approach to treatment; there does not appear to be any medical or surgical treatment that can reverse ovarian ageing. There have been anecdotal reports of spontaneous remission and pregnancy in some females with the so-called resistant ovarian syndrome; but it remains that, anecdotal. Attention should instead be directed towards the management of associated problems such as the multi-system dysfunction that is found in some patients with autoimmune causes of ovarian failure. Furthermore, oestrogen and progesterone replacement therapy should be instituted as soon as possible to prevent the long-term effects of menopause, such as osteoporosis or cardiovascular disease. These problems are most likely to be severe in the patient with ovarian failure occurring at a young age because of the associated long period of resulting oestrogen deficiency.

Women with ovarian failure can still have children but these are generated using donated oocytes. Oocyte donation is now widely practiced in the western world and has resulted in the birth of several thousand children. The donor is usually a young female aged less than 35 years and having had children of her own. Her features should ideally match those of the prospective recipient especially in relation to ethnic background. Although less important, other features such as hair colour, height, build, blood group should match as much as possible. Psychological testing is carried out and in-depth counselling is performed. These are aimed at ascertaining the suitability of the parties concerned and making sure that they are aware of both short- and long-term psychological and social consequences of procreation with donated gametes. Anonymous donation is most ideal and should be aimed for; the donor will however, never know if viable pregnancies and children were generated with her oocytes, or the identity of the children and their subsequent progress in life.

The actual treatment is similar to that described in later chapters for assisted conception. In vitro fertilization (IVF) is carried out using oocytes retrieved from the donor's ovaries and sperm produced by the recipient's husband. A selected number of resulting embryos is transferred into the recipient's uterus two to five days following the oocyte retrieval procedure. Prior to this time the recipient's endometrium is primed to receive and nurture the embryos by the use of oestradiol tablets for about 14 days followed by the administration of progesterone pessaries for two to five days (depending on the age of the embryos) before the embryo transfer. Administration of oestrogen and progesterone is continued until 8–12 weeks of pregnancy, for those who succeed in becoming pregnant. Interestingly, pregnancy rates following IVF using donated oocytes are generally high; often higher than rates obtained in women with normal ovarian function who use their own oocytes for IVF treatment. Oocyte donation may be the only way in which a couple can have children as stipulated requirements for adoption in many countries often do not favour such couples. Although the resulting child will only be genetically related to the recipient's husband the experience of pregnancy by the woman is no different from that of spontaneously conceiving women or those who become pregnant following assisted conception treatment with their own oocytes. Furthermore, this confers motherhood on the recipient, albeit gestational.

Antisperm antibodies in the female

The clinical management of females with antisperm antibodies has not been encouraging. The use of condoms by the man for six to nine months has been tried in an attempt to ascertain if non-contact with semen will lead to a fall in antibody titre in sensitized females with a consequent increase of pregnancy rates following resumption of unprotected sexual intercourse. This has not been found to be the case (Kremer, 1979). Immunosuppressive treatment using steroids in the female has been tried with mixed results but the overwhelming experience has been that this does not lead to a reduction in the antibody level that translates to an improved pregnancy rate. If treatment is required for infertility the couple are best advised to

Table 7.3. Medical management of endometriosis

Combined oral contraceptive pills (contain oestrogen and progesterone)

Progestogens such as medroxyprogesterone acetate, norethindrone acetate, norgestrel acetate and lynestrol

Methyltestosterone

Danazol

Gestrinone

Gonadotrophin releasing hormone agonists such as leuprolide, nafarelin and buserelin

Mifepristone (RU486)

have intrauterine insemination (IUI) (Chapter 12) or IVF treatment (Chapters 8 and 9).

Vaginismus

Psychotherapy is the mainstay of treatment in these couples. Depending on the technique being used, an attempt is made to determine if there is something in the female's past that caused or contributed to the problem. The present union is also examined carefully. Sexual therapy is incorporated into the treatment at some stage later on and will include the woman being encouraged to insert graduated dilators into the vagina while learning to relax the vaginal walls. Eventually, she will try to allow insertion of the penis and hopefully sexual intercourse. Vaginismus may be intractable in some cases and defies treatment. If the couple are still keen to have children, IUI (Meniru et al., 1997) or IVF can be carried out, although she may require some form of anaesthesia or analgesia to allow the required vaginal instrumentation.

Endometriosis

The management of endometriosis in an infertile patient is quite different from that of other women, especially those who have completed their family or do not wish to have children in the immediate future; the treatment should neither worsen the infertile state nor prolong the period of infertility.

Medical treatment of endometriosis has been a traditional modality and various agents that have been used are shown in Table 7.3. The use of these regimens devolve from the fact that endometriotic tissue is hormone dependant. Endometriotic tissue has been shown to contain receptors for oestrogen, progesterone and androgens. Stimulation by oestrogen encourages growth of the endometriotic tissue while androgens have an opposite effect, inducing atrophy of the tissue. Progesterone may stimulate growth of endometriotic tissue but the synthetic progesterone preparations that are used in treating endometriosis usually have androgenic properties and this eventually leads to atrophy of the tissue. In addition to these direct effects on endometriotic tissue most medical treatment aims to suppress ovulation when administered long enough and at a high enough dosage thereby inducing an oestrogen deficiency state akin to that of menopause. This leads to the atrophy of endometriotic tissue due to a lack of significant oestrogenic stimulation.

Surgical treatment aims at excision of endometriotic tissue, including endometrioma, release of adhesions and repair of associated damage to pelvic organs. For amenable females, especially those who are above 40 years of age, removal of both ovaries is carried out together with the fallopian tubes (bilateral salpingo-oophorectomy), and possibly the uterus (hysterectomy). Bilateral oophorectomy removes the oestrogenic stimulus leading to atrophy of endometriotic tissue. Such women, however, will have troublesome menopausal symptoms but current evidence suggests that hormone replacement therapy using weak oestrogenic agents will abolish these symptoms without causing regrowth of the endometriotic tissue.

Further details of medical and surgical treatment of endometriosis will not be provided in this chapter as they have been amply discussed in eminent gynaecology texts. Moreover, a clear distinction was not made, in the past, between the management of infertile women who are found to have endometriosis and other women in whom either conception was not of immediate concern or they did not wish to have any(more) children in future. The aim of treatment in the latter group of women is usually to stop pain and associated symptoms, and is invariably contraceptive during the medical treatment period (six to nine months). Surgical treatment including removal of both ovaries will be required in some of the women.

This does not necessarily mean that medical and surgical treatment of endometriosis has no role in infertility management. However, the traditional approach to the treatment of endometriosis which prolongs the state of infertility or involves major pelvic surgery, albeit often laparoscopic nowadays, without any guarantee of restoration of fertility at the end of the treatment is no more acceptable. As has been stressed in other chapters the age of the woman is crucial and no aspect of infertility management should be allowed to waste her remaining period of optimal fertility. The type of management adopted towards infertility in a couple in which the woman is shown to have endometriosis will depend on the couple's response to the following questions which are repeated in various sections of this book and have been discussed by Jansen (1995): (1) how long have the couple been trying for a pregnancy; (2) how much longer do the couple wish to continue trying; (3) how old is the woman; and (4) can the couple afford assisted conception treatment.

A few examples will be given to illustrate the application of this concept to the management of endometriosis in infertile couples. A couple who have been trying to achieve pregnancy for eight years and the woman is shown to have mild to minimal endometriosis, will not be helped in any way at all by the current debate regarding the uncertain relationship of this degree of endometriosis and the presence of infertility. In the same vein medical or surgical treatment of the endometriosis is not a reasonable option. Such a couple should ideally have assisted conception treatment with IUI or preferably IVF. The presence of moderate to severe endometriosis in another patient who is aged 39 years should also be disregarded and IVF treatment offered. However, pre-treatment with GnRH agonists for two to three months may be suggested as this seems to have a beneficial effect on the outcome of IVF treatment in patients with such a degree of endometriosis. Laparoscopic resection may be the best option for a couple who have been trying for one year to achieve a pregnancy and the woman is aged 25 years with moderately severe endometriosis; they usually do not wish to have assisted conception treatment until they have tried more traditional treatments.

Endometriosis is a chronic disease and tends to recur after treatment unless natural or surgically induced menopause supervenes. It is a truism that the relationship of the disease and infertility is often nebulous. This underscores the importance of treating infertility rather than trying to eliminate endometriotic lesions as there is no assurance that the latter treatment will aid conception.

Tubal problems

The presence of adhesions around the fallopian tubes (peritubal adhesions) and blockage of the tubes are two problems that will be considered here. The advent of assisted conception treatments, notably IVF, has led to a de-emphasis on the use of surgery to correct damaged tubes. This is due to the poor results that follow tubal surgery in general. Some workers believe it is more cost-effective to treat patients with tubal problems using IVF rather than attempting surgical correction while others believe otherwise. The major argument in favour of tubal surgery is that successful correction of a tubal problem makes it possible for the woman to become pregnant any number of times she wishes. This is in contrast to the patient who does not have surgery, instead relying on IVF to achieve conception; it may take several attempts for this to happen thereby incurring heavy financial and other costs. In modern reproductive surgery all attempts are made to identify those women who will benefit from surgery and those who will not. The latter group are offered IVF treatment as the first choice.

Factors that determine the outcome following tubal surgery include the degree and location of the tubal damage. Good prognosis patients for tubal surgery include those with few fine filmy adhesions and patent fallopian tubes; such patients may have cumulative conception rates approaching 60% at two years following surgery (Balen & Jacobs, 1997). Those with dense peritubal adhesions have a much poorer prognosis. This is irrespective of the fact that the adhesions can be divided surgically because adhesions tend to reform. On a similar note females with localized tubal damage such as is seen following conservative tubal sterilization procedures have a much better chance of successful surgical correction than those whose tubal blockage is as a result of diffuse damage along the fallopian tube as is common after chronic or recurrent tubal infections. Other factors such as the age of the woman, duration of infertility and the co-existence of other infertility problems can also influence the decision on whether to attempt tubal surgery or to have IVF treatment.

Two surgical approaches are used for tubal reconstructive surgery. In the open approach the abdomen is opened with a relatively large incision allowing direct access to the pelvic organs. While naked eye visualization was used in the past (macrosurgery) operating microscopes or magnifying binocular loupes are normally used nowadays to aid visualization of the pelvic organs and ensure the correct apposition of the tissue layers during suturing (microsurgery). Other safeguards that are adopted to reduce damage to tissues include using specially designed non-traumatic instruments, continuous irrigation of the exposed pelvic organs to prevent desiccation of their delicate lining membranes, minimal handling of tissues, sealing all bleeding points, leaving no raw surfaces on the organs, use of antibiotics and the use of anti-inflammatory agents including steroids to decrease the risk of adhesion formation following surgery. The suture materials are usually inert and non-absorbable such as nylon although some practitioners use absorbable sutures like vicryl (Balen & Jacobs, 1997). Adhesion barriers are still being evaluated. These are materials that can be used to cover raw surfaces following pelvic surgery in an attempt to reduce the incidence and severity of adhesion formation.

The second approach to tubal surgery that has become popular in recent years is laparoscopy. Operating instruments are introduced into the abdomen through tiny incisions in the abdominal wall. Three to four portals of entry into the abdomen may be required. Visualization of the operating field is by the use of a high definition camera that is mounted on the laparoscope and the image is displayed on monitors that are placed at convenient locations in the operating room. A number of tissue cutting tools can be used including tiny scissors, diathermy, lasers and ultrasonic scalpels. The latter three tools also have the capability to seal bleeding points while cutting; ligatures or metal clips can be placed around larger bleeding points or on good calibre blood vessels before they are cut. Pelvic irrigation is carried out as mentioned above and similar ancillary measures are taken in an attempt to reduce the likelihood of adhesion formation following surgery. The major advantage of the laparoscopic approach lies in the fact that the patient is able to go home on that same day or the following one thereby saving costs. The convalescence period is also shorter and post-operative morbidity (ill health) less.

The major tubal surgical procedures are adhesiolysis (salpingolysis), salpingostomy, resection and tubal reanastomosis, and tubal implantation. Peritubal adhesions are divided during salpingolysis as already described. In salpingostomy a blocked tube is opened with an incision that is made at the side (linear salpingostomy) or at the end (terminal salpingostomy). When only a discrete portion of the tube is blocked but with the ends open, the blocked portion can be cut off (resected) and the tube rejoined (reanastomosis). Tubal blockage close to the uterus or in the portion of the tube that lies within the uterine wall can be treated by resecting the tube just prior to the block and re-implanting the cut end of the tube in a hole that is made in the uterine wall. A less traumatic way of managing this variety of (proximal) tubal blockage is by inserting guide wires into the tube from the uterine cavity and passing graduated dilators (or an inflatable balloon type device) to open up the blocked segment. Finally, there is a relatively high incidence of ectopic pregnancy of 3–10% following tubal surgery. This makes it mandatory for any woman who becomes pregnant following tubal surgery to have early investigations to check for this problem. Such investigations include measurement of the concentration of progesterone, serial quantitative assays of β-hCG in the blood and early (five weeks gestation) transvaginal ultrasound scans to check for the presence of an intrauterine gestation sac.

Conclusion

The advent of assisted reproduction technology has led to the discontinuation of ineffective medical and surgical treatment modalities for infertility and a refining of the criteria for the application of the remaining treatment options. This in no way detracts from the importance of these traditional treatments. Rather it allows their selective application in situations where they have been documented to be effective. This is in contrast to their previous empirical use. Medical and surgical treatments still have important roles in the management of infertility.

BIBLIOGRAPHY

Balen, A. H. & Jacobs, H. S. (1997). *Infertility in Practice*. New York: Churchill Livingstone.

British National Formulary (1999). London: British Medical Association and Royal Pharmaceutical Society of Great Britain.

Crich, J. P. & Jequier, A. M. (1978). Infertility in men with retrograde ejaculation: the action of urine on sperm motility and a simple method for achieving antegrade ejaculation. *Fertility and Sterility* **30**, 572–6.

Derry, F. A., Dinsmore, W. W., Fraser, M. et al. (1998). Efficacy and safety of oral sildenafil (Viagra) in men with erectile dysfunction caused by spinal cord injury. *Neurology* **51**, 1629–33.

Droegemueller, W. (1997). Endometriosis and adenomyosis. In *Comprehensive Gynecology*, ed. D. R. Mishell, M. A. Stenchever, W. Droegemueller & A. L. Herbst, pp. 517–46. New York: Mosby.

Ginsburg, J., Hardiman, P. & Thomas, M. (1992). Vaginal bromocriptine: clinical and biochemical effects. *Gynecological Endocrinology* **6**, 119–26.

Jansen, R. P. (1995). Elusive fertility: fecundability and assisted conception in perspective. *Fertility and Sterility* **64**, 252–4.

Kloner, R. A. (1998). Viagra: what every physician should know. *Ear, Nose and Throat Journal* **77**, 783–6.

Kremer, J. (1979). A new technique for intrauterine insemination. *International Journal of Fertility* **24**, 53–6.

Marshburn, P. B. & Kutteh, W. H. (1994). The role of antisperm antibodies in infertility. *Fertility and Sterility* **61**, 799–811.

Meniru, G. I., Brinsden, P. R. & Craft, I. L. (1997). *A Handbook of Intrauterine Insemination.* Cambridge: Cambridge University Press.

Mishell, D. R. Jr. (1997). Hyperprolactinaemia, galactorrhea, and pituitary adenomas. In *Comprehensive Gynecology*, ed. D. R. Mishell, M. A. Stenchever, W. Droegemueller & A. L. Herbst, pp. 1069–86. New York: Mosby.

Morales, A., Gingell, C., Collins, M. et al. (1998). Clinical safety of oral sildenafil citrate (Viagra) in the treatment of erectile dysfunction. *International Journal of Impotence Research* **10**, 69–73.

Schlaff, W. D. & Kletzky, O. A. (1998). Amenorrhea, hyperprolactinemia, and chronic anovulation. In *Essentials of Obstetrics and Gynecology*, ed. N. F. Hacker & J. G. Moore, 3rd edn, pp. 580–93. Philadelphia: W. B. Saunders Company.

Speroff, L., Glass, R. H. & Kase, N. G. (1999). *Clinical Gynecologic Endocrinology and Infertility*, 6th edn. Baltimore: Lippincott Williams & Wilkins.

Tan, S. L. & Jacobs, H. S. (1991). *Infertility, Your Questions Answered.* Singapore: McGraw-Hill Book Co.

Vermesh, M., Fossum, G. T. & Kletzky, O. A. (1988). Vaginal bromocriptine: pharmacology and effect on serum prolactin in normal women. *Obstetrics and Gynecology* **72**, 693–8.

Viera, A. J., Clenney, T. L., Shenenberger, D. W. & Green, G. F. (1999). Newer pharmacologic alternatives for erectile dysfunction. *American Family Physician* **60**, 1159–72.

Zippe, C. D., Kedia, A. W., Kedia, K. et al. (1998). Treatment of erectile dysfunction after radical prostatectomy with sildenafil citrate (Viagra). *Urology* **52**, 963–6.

8

Conventional in vitro fertilization treatment

Introduction

The first birth in 1978 following in vitro fertilization (IVF) treatment (Steptoe & Edwards, 1978) marked the beginning of a rapid expansion of treatment modalities available to infertile couples as well as an improvement in success rates. IVF and many other assisted conception treatments are now routinely carried out in clinical practice and are proving to be more efficient and cost effective than some traditional medical remedies, such as tubal surgery for example, in certain classes of patients. Conventional IVF is the name given to the original 'test tube baby' treatment method and involves addition of a measured volume of prepared sperm suspension to a dish containing the retrieved oocytes. Most other variants of conventional IVF still share several similarities with it. Where they differ is mainly in the method used to procure fertilization of the oocytes and the site of deposition of the gametes or embryos in the female genital tract. The various stages of conventional IVF treatment will now be described. Other assisted conception treatment methods will be described in subsequent chapters. It is important that practical information similar to that contained in the following account is made available to infertile couples by their carers. Couples who are aware of all aspects of their treatment will be more co-operative since they know exactly what to expect and when. Most importantly they are fully informed on issues such as success rates of the treatment, complications and possible side-effects.

Patient selection for conventional IVF and related treatments

When is conventional IVF the treatment of choice for couples with infertility and what are the indications? The answer to this question is multifaceted although actually very simple. The first requirement is the decision to have assisted conception treatment. The potential candidates are those who have been trying unsuccessfully for a pregnancy for more than two years, who have the financial resources for assisted conception treatment and have made up their mind to have the treatment before the woman's age becomes an additional obstacle to success. Those women with failing ovarian function by reason of older age or other causes, can still have conventional IVF treatment but with donor oocytes. The next stage in the decision-making process is to exclude factors that reduce the efficacy of the proposed treatment and offer affected patients alternative treatment options that have a better chance of succeeding. For example, conventional IVF is not a suitable treatment for patients with azoospermia or severe oligo-, astheno- and/or teratozoospermia. These patients are best treated with intracytoplasmic sperm injection (Chapter 9) which may involve surgical sperm retrieval (Chapter 10). For the remaining couples, it has to be decided if conventional IVF should be offered as a first option or when more traditional medical and surgical remedies, and less invasive or expensive assisted conception treatment options fail. Those patients in whom IVF is offered as a second option have the greatest risk of being mismanaged. Such patients may spend years being administered ineffective treatment and by the time they reach the stage of having IVF treatment they are much older and there will be a greater concern with female age-related reproductive dysfunction than before. It is probably better to err on the side of early recourse to assisted conception treatment, with conventional IVF, than a late decision to do so provided the couple can afford the cost of the treatment. There is now a greater realization that conventional IVF and related treatment techniques are more effective than some traditional medical and surgical remedies, especially in well chosen cases. These considerations are illustrated in Figure 8.1. IVF treatment has now evolved to the point where it can be confidently offered as a first line treatment modality irrespective of the primary cause of infertility, provided the said cause does not contraindicate the use of IVF treatment as already discussed above. Finally, IVF is the ultimate diagnostic test of the procreative ability of the couple and can provide valuable insight into the causation of infertility in a couple, more than can be gained by using the investigations discussed in Chapter 6. Thus, it is not uncommon to find unexpected problems arising during IVF treatment such as listed in Table 8.1. Although the origin of some of these problems may lie in the treatment technique used, for example polyspermic fertilization arising from the use of a high insemination concentration of sperm, others cannot be so easily explained away; they probably have a bearing on how the state of infertility arose in the couple.

Manipulation of the menstrual cycle

In large assisted conception units, treatment of infertile couples takes place on virtually everyday of the week (Ben-Chetrit et al., 1997). As such it does not matter what phase of the menstrual cycle the individual patients are in; administration of the various medications to each patient is commenced and conducted without

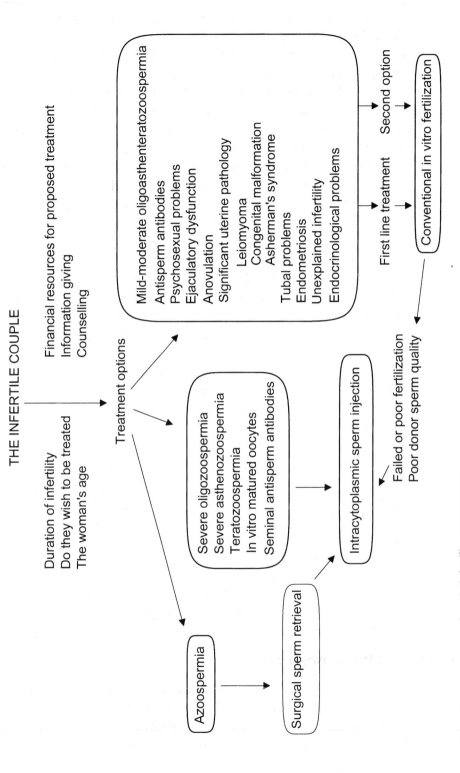

Figure 8.1 Decision-making in infertility management.

Table 8.1. Unexpected problems noted during in vitro fertilization treatment that may have a bearing on the causation of the couples' infertility

---

Poor ovarian response to superovulation in the presence of normal blood concentrations of
    FSH and LH
Complete fertilization failure
Poor fertilization rate
Single pronucleus
Polyspermic fertilization
Predominance of poor quality oocytes in the retrieved cohort
Predominance of abnormal oocytes in the retrieved cohort
Predominance of poor quality embryos
Poor in vitro embryo development

Notes: FSH: follicle stimulating hormone; LH: luteinizing hormone.

much reference to other patients in the unit. The situation is different in smaller units where it is more cost-effective to group patients together and run cycles of treatment at set times during the year (Egbase et al., 1996). Not every woman will be at the required phase of the menstrual cycle at these times. Therefore, there may be a need to readjust the menstrual cycles of such women to make it possible for all patients to commence ovarian stimulation at the required time. The manipulation of menstrual cycles involves the use of progestogens such as medroxyprogesterone acetate, dydrogesterone and norethindrone (Engmann et al., 1999) or oral contraceptive tablets. These can either be used to postpone the onset of the next menstrual period or bring it forward. Some patients may not need these medications since they will already be at the right phase of the menstrual period.

Gonadotrophin releasing hormone agonists (GnRHa)

These drugs are used to prevent the pituitary gland from interfering with the function of the ovaries during ovarian stimulation. Normally, the pituitary gland controls ovarian function in humans such that only one oocyte is ovulated in each ovarian cycle. During IVF treatment, the ovaries are stimulated with relatively large doses of follicle stimulating hormone (FSH) and luteinizing hormone (LH) which are administered as daily injections. This is aimed at the production of many (5–20) oocytes. This approach to ovarian stimulation is called superovulation and is distinct from ovulation induction (described in Chapter 7) which aims at the production of just one oocyte similar to the usual situation in nature.

The pituitary gland normally stimulates the release of the mature oocyte by suddenly increasing the production of LH towards midcycle. This natural LH surge

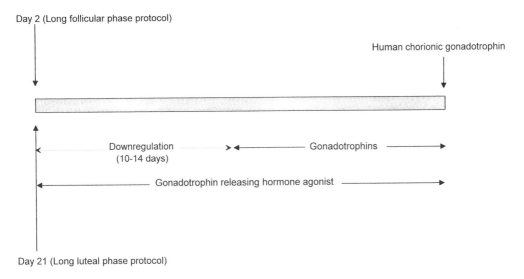

Day 2 (Long follicular phase protocol)

Human chorionic gonadotrophin

Downregulation
(10–14 days)

Gonadotrophins

Gonadotrophin releasing hormone agonist

Day 21 (Long luteal phase protocol)

Figure 8.2   The long protocols of pituitary desensitization.

which occurs about 36–40 hours before ovulation is undesirable during IVF treatment for three reasons: (1) it may occur prematurely before an adequate number of oocytes reach the required stage of development; (2) the endogenous output of LH may not be adequate for the induction of final maturational changes in all the developing oocytes; and (3) since the oocytes have to be aspirated from the ovaries before ovulation occurs, it is important that events are programmed such that ovulation does not occur before medical staff are ready for the oocyte aspiration procedure.

GnRHa are analogues of gonadotrophin releasing hormone (GnRH) but are several times more powerful. Their administration causes a high output of FSH and LH from the pituitary gland but this is relatively short lasting. Continued administration of GnRHa depletes the pituitary stores of these hormones and their output falls to very low levels. This is called pituitary downregulation and the lack of response of the pituitary gland to further doses of GnRHa is said to be due to pituitary desensitization. These events are usually completed within 10–14 days of starting chronic GnRHa administration. Gonadotrophin releasing hormone *antagonists* have now been developed (Lin et al., 1999; Rongieres-Bertrand et al., 1999) and just entered clinical practice. The first available preparations are ganirelix acetate and cetrorelix acetate. These antagonists act by immediately suppressing pituitary output of FSH and LH without causing the initial flare up of the production of these hormones unlike GnRHa.

There are three established methods of administering GnRHa during superovulation and they have been given the name 'protocols' (Figures 8.2 and 8.3). In the

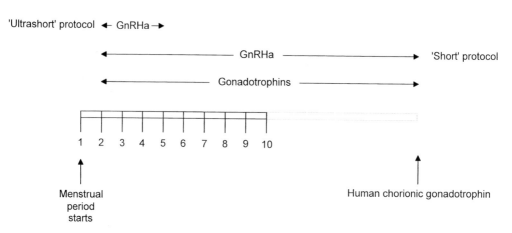

Figure 8.3   The short and ultrashort protocols of pituitary desensitization.

'long protocol' GnRHa administration is commenced from either the midluteal phase (Day 21) of the menstrual cycle preceding the treatment cycle or from the early follicular phase (Day 2) of the treatment cycle itself. The GnRHa is administered for 10–14 days before commencing the injection of gonadotrophins and continued until the administration of the ovulation trigger. The 'short protocol' involves the use of GnRHa from Days 1, 2, or 3 of the treatment cycle until the day of administration of the ovulation trigger. Gonadotrophin injections are commenced one or two days after starting GnRHa administration. In the 'ultrashort protocol' GnRHa administration is commenced on Days 1, 2 or 3 of the treatment cycle but is limited to just three days. It is believed that this disrupts pituitary production of FSH and LH long enough to complete superovulation and administer the ovulation trigger. However, there is a higher incidence of premature LH surge compared to the other protocols. The long protocol is the most popular protocol of GnRHa administration and the ultrashort protocol is least used.

A list of available GnRHa is given in Table 8.2. Buserelin is one of the commonly used drugs and is normally administered as an intranasal spray. The drug is sprayed into one of the nostrils four to five times a day. A convenient schedule is 7 a.m., 11 a.m., 3 p.m., 7 p.m. and 11 p.m. Buserelin can also be administered as an injection once a day. Nafarelin has a more convenient twice daily intranasal administration schedule and it is easier to ensure patient compliance with this than with Buserelin. Nafarelin is administered into each nostril twice daily although some clinicians prescribe its administration into only one nostril twice daily. Prostap SR, Lupron Depot and Zoladex only need to be administered once; the injections are made into the subcutaneous fat of the anterior abdominal wall below the umbilicus. The application of a generous amount of local anaesthetic cream on the skin,

Table 8.2. Gonadotrophin releasing hormone agonists

Agonist	Brand name	Manufacturer	Route of administration
Buserelin	Suprecur	Hoechst	N
	Suprefact	Hoechst	N/SC
Goserelin	Zoladex	ICI	SC-implant
Leuprorelin	Prostap SR	Lederle-Takeda	SC/IM
	Lucrin	Abbott	SC
Leuprolide	Lupron Depot	TAP	IM
Naferelin	Synarel	Syntex	N
Triptorelin	Decapeptyl	Salk/Ferring	SC-implant

Notes: SC: subcutaneous; IM: intramuscular; N: intranasal.

and covering it with a non-porous non-absorbent dressing, two hours before the injection largely eliminates the pain caused by piercing the skin with the relatively large bore needle that is attached to the pre-filled pre-packed injection kit. One administration of these depot GnRHa preparations lasts for about 28 days. If GnRHa action is required for longer than this period, intranasal or daily injections of GnRHa preparations are given on those extra days.

Suppression of pituitary activity will be required for about four weeks (28 days) generally. In some cases GnRHa may be given for longer than 10–14 days before starting gonadotrophin injections. This happens when it is difficult to programme the menstrual cycle of some patients with Provera, Duphaston, oral contraceptive tablets or similar medication. The GnRHa is continued for 21, 28 or any number of days required to get the woman into the right stage for gonadotrophin injections to be started. In other women, pituitary suppression may not be achieved within the usual time frame or cysts may form in their ovaries following commencement of GnRHa administration. Such women are maintained on GnRHa for a longer time and in the latter case long enough to allow the cysts to regress completely. In fact, women who have been having GnRHa treatment for endometriosis, usually for three to six months, can even start IVF treatment without waiting for the normal menstrual periods to return (Edwards et al., 1996).

Superovulation

Ovarian stimulation for IVF treatment aims for multiple follicular development and the retrieval of many oocytes. It is believed that the chances of conception are improved by the transfer of more than one good quality embryo into the uterine cavity (Meniru & Craft, 1997). Table 8.3 shows various superovulation regimens that have been used in the past or are currently being used by different assisted

Table 8.3. Ovarian cycle management for in vitro fertilization

Natural cycle
Clomiphene citrate
Clomiphene citrate + hMG
Clomiphene citrate + FSH
hMG
FSH
hMG + FSH
GnRHa + hMG
GnRHa + FSH
GnRHa + hMG + FSH
GnRHa + rFSH

Notes: FSH: follicle stimulating hormone; GnRHa: gonadotrophin releasing hormone agonist; hMG: human menopausal gonadotrophin; rFSH: recombinant follicle stimulating hormone.

Table 8.4. Gonadotrophin preparations

Gonadotrophin	Brands	Company
hMG	Humegon (FSH:LH = 1:1)	Organon
	Normegon (FSH:LH = 3:1)	Organon
	Pergonal (FSH:LH = 1:1)	Serono
'Pure' FSH	Metrodin, Metrodin "High" Purity	Serono
	Orgafol	Organon
hCG	Gonadotraphon	Paines & Byrne
	Pregnyl	Organon
	Profasi	Serono
Recombinant FSH	Gonal-F	Serono
	Puregon	Organon

Notes: FSH: follicle stimulating hormone; hMG: human menopausal gonadotrophin; hCG: human chorionic gonadotrophin.

conception units (Pados et al., 1995). Clomiphene citrate was used initially, with or without gonadotrophin injections, for ovarian stimulation. Most units now use a combination of GnRHa and gonadotrophin injections. Various brands of gonadotrophins are available (Table 8.4). Some contain mainly FSH while others contain a mixture of LH and FSH (Weissman, 1999). Initially these gonadotrophin preparations were produced by extraction of FSH and LH from the urine of postmenopausal women. However, in recent years two preparations (Gonal F and Puregon – Follistim in the USA) have come into clinical use and are produced using recombinant DNA technology.

Gonadotrophin injections

The dose of gonadotrophin injection administered to any particular patient depends on factors such as age, build, dose used in previous treatment cycles, whether the ovaries are polycystic, history of ovarian hyperstimulation syndrome (OHSS) in a previous treatment cycle and ovarian or periovarian surgery. The dose may have to be increased or decreased depending on her response to the administered drugs. Some patients may receive 100–150 IU a day while others will receive 225 IU or more. A successful treatment outcome becomes less common when more than 450 IU are required each day especially when there is evidence of incipient ovarian failure in the pre-treatment period. Gonadotrophin injections are continued until many of the developing follicles attain the diameter of 18–22 mm. The injections are usually given for a total of 12–16 days but administration can be extended to 21 days for poor responders or when there is a very cautious approach to superovulation, for example, in those who had a previous OHSS or are known to have polycystic ovaries.

Ovulation triggers

Since the natural LH surge is abolished by the use of GnRHa, alternative ovulation triggers are required. The LH surge initiates final maturation of the oocyte and softening of connective tissue elements that anchor the oocyte–cumulus complex (OCC) to the wall of the follicle. The latter change makes it easier for the OCC to become dislodged at the time of ovulation or oocyte aspiration. Human chorionic gonadotrophin (hCG) is a glycoprotein hormone that shares key structural similarities with LH and can induce similar oocyte maturation in developing follicles. An injection of 5000–10 000 IU of the drug is administered when the developing follicles reach the required size. The oocytes are aspirated from the ovaries about 34–36 hours after the hCG injection. The brand names of commonly used hCG preparations are A.P.L., Pregnyl and Profasi. The administration of GnRHa is stopped once hCG is injected.

If GnRHa is not administered for pituitary down-regulation and desensitization it can be used at midcycle to stimulate an upsurge of LH and FSH production by the pituitary. An example is Buserelin which can be administered subcutaneously as a single dose of 1 mg. The resulting output of LH and FSH stimulates final developmental changes as detailed above.

Ultrasound scans

Ultrasound scanning is the main method of monitoring the woman's response to ovarian stimulation. Most of the scanning will be carried out transvaginally

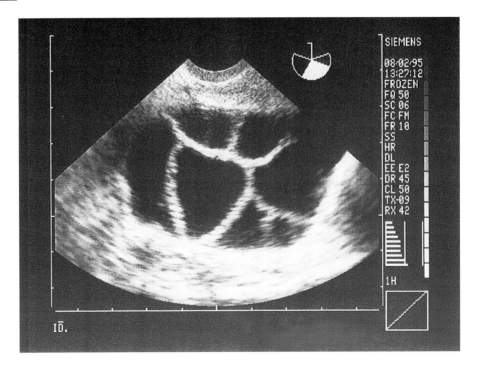

Figure 8.4   Transvaginal sonogram: developing follicles in the ovary during superovulation.

because this gives the best image of the pelvic organs as it allows the use of higher ultrasound frequencies. The ultrasound probe is covered with one or two disposable rubber sheaths before being gently introduced into the vagina and used to scan the pelvis. The probe is washed and sterilized by dipping it into glutaraldhyde solution for up to 20–30 minutes in between patients or at the end of the working day.

An initial ultrasound scan is carried out 10–14 days after commencing GnRHa treatment. The endometrial lining is examined to make sure it is thin and normal. The endometrial thickness is preferably less than 3 mm and should not measure more than 5 mm. The ovaries are carefully examined to exclude cysts or any other abnormalities. As noted earlier in this chapter the initial flare-up of FSH and LH production after commencing GnRHa administration may lead to the formation of a follicular cyst. The cyst can either be left alone or aspirated before commencing gonadotrophin administration. Alternatively the GnRHa can be continued until the cyst disappears before commencing gonadotrophin administration.

The next ultrasound scan will be scheduled to take place after six to eight days of gonadotrophin injections. Subsequently, scans are carried out daily, every other day or at longer intervals depending on the observed patient response. On each occasion the ovaries and uterus are examined. The number of developing follicles in

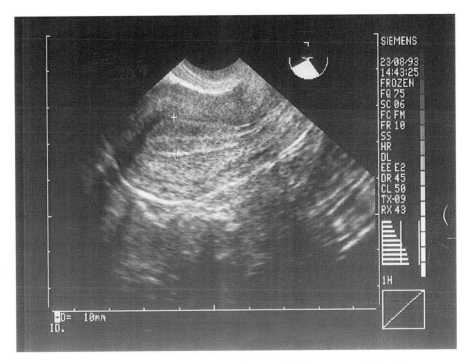

Figure 8.5 Transvaginal sonogram: the endometrium exhibits a triple line pattern during the proliferative phase of the menstrual or superovulated cycle. The central line marks the endometrial cavity.

each ovary is checked and their size measured (Figure 8.4). The endometrial thickness and reflectivity are assessed and noted (Figures 8.5 and 8.6).

Hormone assays

The concentration of oestrogen, progesterone, FSH and LH may be measured through blood tests that are carried out 10–14 days after commencing GnRHa treatment. This is to ensure that adequate control has been achieved over pituitary function. Subsequent hormone assays measure mainly oestrogen which is produced by the developing follicles in the ovaries. The concentration of this hormone in blood can give an indication of how well the ovaries are responding to the stimulation and whether the woman is over responding to the gonadotrophin injections. It may be useful to include LH as one of the hormones the concentration of which is assayed in the latter part of the treatment cycle, especially in women who are on the ultrashort protocol, to detect any premature rise in the concentration of the hormone. It is not uncommon to note a rise in progesterone concentration in the latter part of the stimulation phase of the cycle in some patients. This

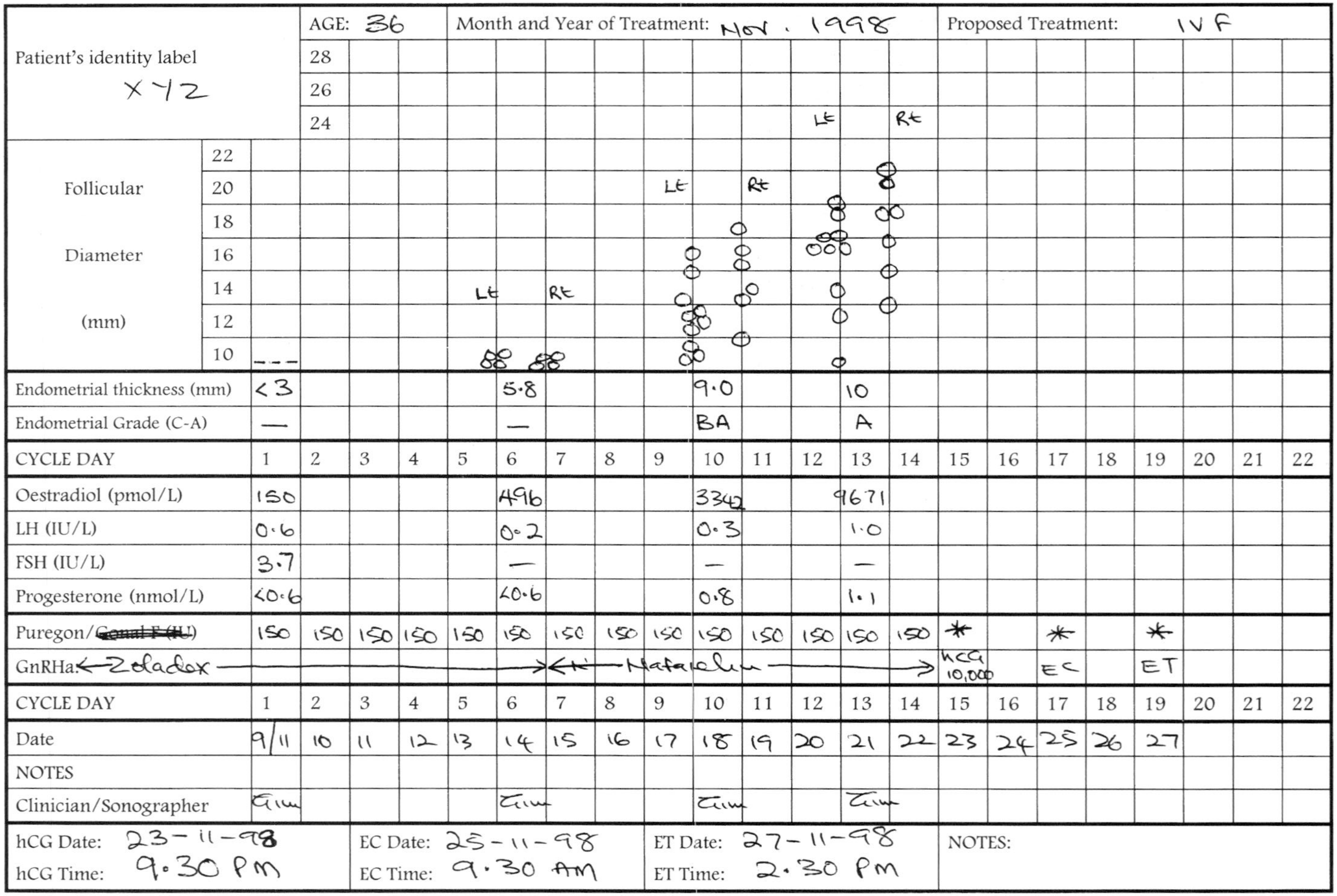

Patient's identity label: X/2

AGE: 36 Month and Year of Treatment: Nov. 1998 Proposed Treatment: IVF

Follicular Diameter (mm): 28, 26, 24, 22, 20, 18, 16, 14, 12, 10

	1	2	3	4	5	6	7	8	9	10	11	12	13	14	15	16	17	18	19	20	21	22
Endometrial thickness (mm)	<3					5.8				9.0			10									
Endometrial Grade (C–A)	–					–				BA			A									
CYCLE DAY	1	2	3	4	5	6	7	8	9	10	11	12	13	14	15	16	17	18	19	20	21	22
Oestradiol (pmol/L)	150					496				334			9671									
LH (IU/L)	0.6					0.2				0.3			1.0									
FSH (IU/L)	3.7					–				–			–									
Progesterone (nmol/L)	<0.6					<0.6				0.8			1.1									
Puregon	150	150	150	150	150	150	150	150	150	150	150	150	150	150								
GnRHa	←— Nafarelin —→													hCG 10,000	*		*		*			
CYCLE DAY	1	2	3	4	5	6	7	8	9	10	11	12	13	14	15	16	17	18	19	20	21	22
Date	9/11	10	11	12	13	14	15	16	17	18	19	20	21	22	23	24	25	26	27			
NOTES															EC		EC		ET			
Clinician/Sonographer	Tim					Tim				Tim			Tim									

hCG Date: 23-11-98   hCG Time: 9.30 PM
EC Date: 25-11-98   EC Time: 9.30 AM
ET Date: 27-11-98   ET Time: 2.30 PM

NOTES:

Figure 8.6 Folliculogram: a graphical display of follicle number and the pattern of development.

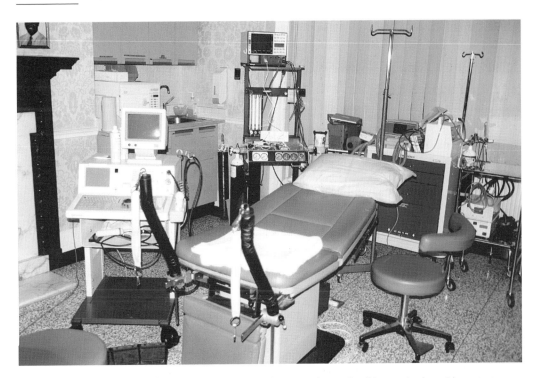

Figure 8.7   A typical procedure room in an assisted conception unit with standard equipment.

premature production of progesterone is not usually as a result of a premature increase in LH production or ovulation and can be noticed even in treatment cycles in which the patient is administered LH-free gonadotrophin preparations such as recombinant FSH. Although an experienced ultrasonographer may suspect the occurrence of this phenomenon by a change in the reflectivity of the endometrium a blood assay of progesterone will make the diagnosis more accurate.

Hormonal assays during ovarian stimulation need not be carried out on every patient or by every unit, since ultrasound scanning often gives sufficient information on which to base a decision on whether to continue superovulation or cancel it (Tsirigotis et al., 1995). However, the availability of information on the blood concentration of these hormones gives more insight into the patient's response. It is also useful in problem patients and for clinic based research.

Oocyte retrieval

The patient reports to the assisted conception unit on the morning of the procedure. She should be fasting for at least five hours; she is usually advised not to have any food or drink from the preceding midnight. She is prepared in the ward and taken to the procedure room of the unit (Figure 8.7). Various forms of anaesthesia

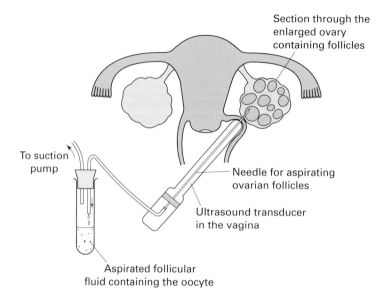

Section through the
enlarged ovary
containing follicles

To suction
pump

Needle for aspirating
ovarian follicles

Ultrasound transducer
in the vagina

Aspirated follicular
fluid containing the oocyte

Figure 8.8 Transvaginal oocyte retrieval.

can be used but short-acting intravenous sedatives and narcotics are popular such
as propofol combined with alfentanil. The vagina can be cleansed with antiseptics
and irrigated with normal saline to remove traces of the antiseptic. There is
however no guarantee that the irrigation will remove all traces of the antiseptic
which if it comes into contact with the oocytes may exert toxic effects. Alternatively,
the vagina can be wiped of all mucus with gauze swabs soaked in normal saline and
no increase in pelvic infection has been noted with this cleaning method especially
if this is performed in conjunction with antibiotic prophylaxis.

A transvaginal ultrasound scan is carried out and oocytes are aspirated from follicles in both ovaries through a needle that is used to pierce the vaginal wall and
puncture the follicle (Figure 8.8). Each tube of aspirated fluid is examined under
magnification (Figure 8.9) to identify the oocyte (Figure 8.10) which is then
removed and washed in clean culture medium. The retrieved oocytes are placed in
culture dishes containing culture medium and kept in an incubator that is maintained at 37°C and having an internal atmosphere of 5–6% CO_2 in humidified air.
Oocytes can also be aspirated from the ovaries during laparoscopy (Figure 8.11).
However, the transvaginal route of oocyte collection that is carried out under
ultrasound guidance is preferred nowadays. Following completion of the oocyte
recovery two suppositories are inserted into the rectum. The first is metronidazole
and it is given (at a dosage of 1 g) just this once for prophylaxis of pelvic infection.
The second suppository is voltarol which provides strong pain relief post-
operatively. The patient can be given alternative antibiotic preparations, that have

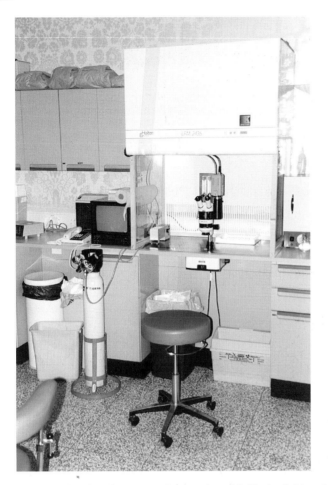

Figure 8.9   The clinical embryologist examines aspirated follicular fluid at this station to identify oocytes.

a wider spectrum of action, such as an intravenous injection of 1.2 g of augmentin.

Transvaginal oocyte collection is a relatively safe procedure. The patient should feel no pain and regain full consciousness soon afterwards. The procedure takes an average of 30 minutes. After a short while in the ward, the patient is usually discharged home on that same day. Before discharge the findings at operation are discussed with the couple and they are informed of the number of oocytes that were collected. The adequacy of the semen sample produced by the man is also confirmed before the couple leave the unit. It is very important that the patient confirms her current phone numbers so that she can be contacted whenever required during the ensuing days. The patient should not drive a vehicle for 24 hours after the procedure. She must be driven home by her partner or a friend.

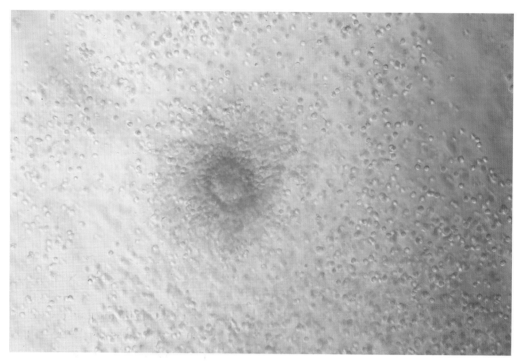

Figure 8.10 Typical appearances of a retrieved oocyte which is usually surrounded by cumulus cells. These cells are dispersed by hyaluronidase enzyme released by spermatozoa in their bid to reach the zona pellucida and fertilize the oocyte.

Production of a semen sample

The patient's partner is required to produce a semen sample. This can be carried out at the same time the oocyte collection is being performed. This arrangement makes it possible for the man to be with his partner until she goes in for the oocyte collection; he then goes and produces the sample and is back before his partner comes out of the procedure room. Alternatively, he can produce the sample before his partner goes in for the oocyte collection especially if there are other patients scheduled to have the procedure before her. The semen sample is generally produced by masturbation following two to three days of abstinence from ejaculation. The quality of the semen sample may become poor if the period of abstinence is more than 7–10 days. The ejaculate is collected into sterile plastic containers which are non-toxic to spermatozoa. It is recommended that the man washes his hands and genitals with soap, rinses them several times with clean water and dries with a clean towel. No lubricant such as petroleum jelly is allowed during masturbation to avoid problems of toxicity to spermatozoa. Other aspects of semen collection have already been described in Chapter 5.

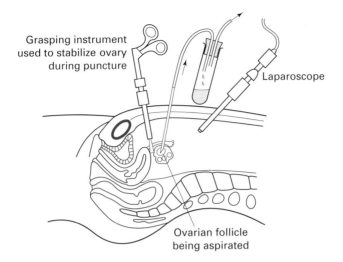

Grasping instrument
used to stabilize ovary
during puncture

Laparoscope

Ovarian follicle
being aspirated

Figure 8.11 Laparoscopically directed oocyte retrieval. This is not commonly performed nowadays.

The semen sample is analysed and then prepared for IVF. Different methods of sperm preparation are in use. All methods aim to remove seminal fluid and its chemical constituents, dead and abnormal spermatozoa and other cells from the sample thereby leaving only normal motile spermatozoa suspended in clean culture medium (Figure 8.12). Rarely, the man may be asked to produce another sample that same morning. This happens when the initial sample is of poor quality and it is hoped that a second sample will be better. This is one of the reasons why the man should not leave the unit without checking with the IVF laboratory to make sure that there is no problem with the semen sample he produced earlier on.

In situations when the man cannot produce a semen sample on demand he is provided with containers to take home. He is asked to masturbate into one of the containers on any day he chooses and bring the sample to the unit. The semen is analysed and frozen for use during future IVF treatment cycles. Obviously, such patients have to be identified beforehand for this strategy to be usefully applied to IVF treatments. If this problem is only detected on the day of oocyte collection one of the options will be to cancel the IVF treatment at that stage. Alternatively, spermatozoa can be aspirated with needles from the man's epididymis and/or testes as described in Chapter 10. The use of donor spermatozoa is the least desired option which should not be readily used nowadays given the availability of techniques for surgical sperm retrieval and electroejaculation. Methods of obtaining semen from men with impotence, retrograde ejaculation and other ejaculatory problems have been described in Chapter 7.

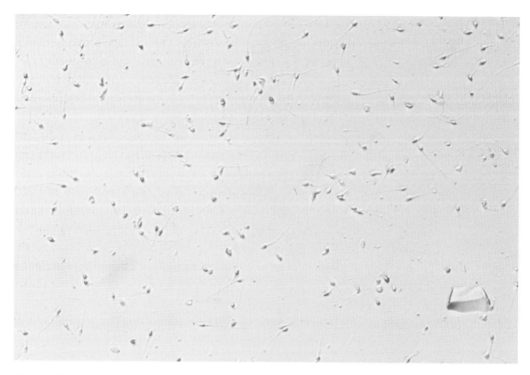

Figure 8.12 Freshly produced semen showing spermatozoa, other cells and debris.

Progesterone supplementation

It is routine for women who have had GnRHa administration to be given progesterone supplementation because it is presently thought these women may not produce enough of the hormone themselves during the luteal phase of that treatment cycle. Normally LH produced by the pituitary supports the development and function of the corpus luteum which produces progesterone in the luteal phase. However, full pituitary recovery following discontinuation of GnRHa administration may take up to 10 days or more. Progesterone supplementation is started in the evening, following oocyte collection or the day after. A commonly used natural progesterone preparation is Cyclogest pessary. A pessary is inserted into the vagina or rectum from where it is absorbed into the blood stream. The dose varies amongst different practitioners. An example is 400 mg inserted twice a day (in the morning and at night; 12 hours apart).

The patient decides whether she wants to insert the pessary in the vagina or rectum. However, she should not insert it into the vagina on the morning of embryo transfer to avoid soiling the vagina with the medication. Insertion of the pessaries is continued until the pregnancy test result is available. If negative, she stops inserting the pessaries; the menstrual period should start within two weeks. If the patient becomes pregnant she continues with progesterone supplementation until 12 weeks of pregnancy. There is no agreement on the ideal regimen to use here. Some practitioners even stop progesterone supplementation once the pregnancy test result is positive while others may prescribe its use for the first six weeks, i.e. up to eight weeks of pregnancy, following embryo transfer.

Another natural progesterone preparation is called Gestone which is in the form of an injection administered by deep intramuscular injection daily. Crinone, a progesterone gel, is a new preparation which can also be used for progesterone supplementation (Pouly et al., 1996). It comes in pre-filled applicators each of which delivers 90 g of progesterone in a small volume of gel. One applicator full of gel is deposited into the vagina once a day. hCG can also be administered to support the function of the corpora lutea, but this is not popular because hCG increases the risk of having OHSS in women who produce several follicles during superovulation. Furthermore, the use of hCG does not seem to confer any advantage over the use of progesterone for luteal support.

Laboratory phase of IVF treatment

On the day of oocyte collection

A measured volume of the prepared sperm suspension is added to the dish containing the oocytes three to six hours after the oocyte collection. The number of inseminated spermatozoa depend on the sperm parameters of the semen sample. Higher numbers will be added to compensate for poorer sperm parameters.

On the day after the oocyte collection

The dish is checked in the morning. Fertilized oocytes are identified and placed in fresh dishes of culture medium and returned to the incubator. Normal fertilization is diagnosed when two pronuclei are seen together with two polar bodies (Figure 8.13). Unfertilized and abnormally fertilized oocytes are discarded. The patient is notified of the fertilization result; normally 40–70% of the oocytes should fertilize. A tentative time the next day is fixed for the embryo replacement.

On the second day after the oocyte collection

The embryos are replaced in the uterus on this day. Embryos can also be replaced on the third, fourth or fifth day. Current research is directed at determining whether embryo replacement on the fifth day confers any advantage over replacement on the other days in the form of an increased pregnancy rate (Gardner et al., 1998a,b). The culture dishes are inspected in the morning to find out which

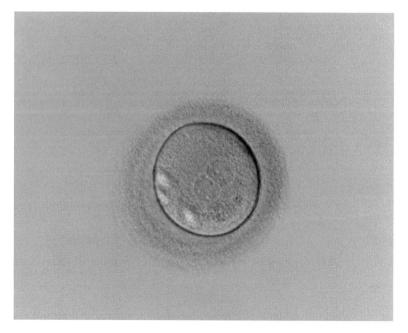

Figure 8.13 Photomicrograph showing a normally fertilized (two-pronuclear) oocyte.

fertilized eggs have started cleaving. Each fertilized egg is expected to have cleaved into two to four cells by this time; all the cells are still enclosed by the zona pellucida. When the fertilized egg starts dividing into cells it is called an embryo. About 90% of fertilized eggs should become embryos. A predetermined number of embryos are selected for replacement in the uterine cavity. Any excess embryos of suitable quality are cryopreserved (frozen). Poor quality embryos are deemed not likely to survive the freezing and thawing process and are discarded.

The number of embryos to replace

This is a contentious issue. It is realized that the chance of pregnancy occurring in any particular patient partly depends on the number of embryos transferred. The more the number of embryos that are transferred the greater the chances of conception, at least up to a certain point. However, the incidence of multiple pregnancy also increases with the number of embryos that are replaced (Devreker et al., 1999; Matson et al., 1999). Up to 25% of pregnancies that occur when three embryos are replaced are twin pregnancies while triplets and higher order multiple pregnancies will be found in about 5–8%. The interrelationship of transferred embryo number with pregnancy and multiple pregnancy rates is shown in Table 8.5. Multiple

Table 8.5. Transferred embryo number and its relationship to pregnancy and multiple pregnancy rates

Number of transferred embryos	Pregnancy rate (%)	Number of fetuses		
		Single (%)	Twin (%)	Triplet or more (%)
1	10	>99	<1	Rare
2	25–30	74	25	1
3	30	70	24	5–8

Notes: The above figures are for illustration purposes. National statistics should be consulted for specific rates for the country concerned.

Table 8.6. Complications of multiple pregnancy

Hyperemesis gravidarum	Pre-eclampsia
Anaemia	Varicose veins
Miscarriage	Polyhydramnios
Fetal malformations	Antepartum haemorrhage
Pedal oedema	Preterm labour and delivery
Dyspepsia	Premature rupture of membranes
Cord accidents	Postpartum haemorrhage
Intrauterine growth retardation	Caesarean delivery
Malpresentation and abnormal lie	Fetal abnormality
Stillbirth	

pregnancy, especially triplet and above, is associated with several complications (Table 8.6).

A compromise which many clinicians generally adopt is to transfer three embryos. Young patients (early to mid-twenties) who are deemed suitable may be advised, but not coerced in any way, to have only two embryos replaced. It is also advisable for females below 35 years of age to have only two embryos replaced the first time they have IVF treatment, provided all other aspects of their treatment are normal. Three embryos may be transferred in women between 36 and 40 years while four embryos may be transferred in women above 40 years, especially if they have had previous unsuccessful treatment. Both the patient and the medical team have to decide on how many embryos to transfer and the patient has the final say on this matter. However, in some countries such as the UK, legislation has limited the number of transferred embryos to a maximum of three. Many IVF centres in

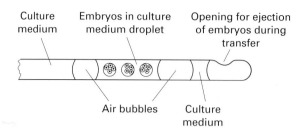

Figure 8.14 Proximal part of an embryo replacement cannula containing embryos in a 10 μl droplet of culture medium that is cushioned by air bubbles and culture medium droplets.

Scandinavia and other countries have now started putting back only two embryos for most patients irrespective of their age, and pregnancy rates have remained good. Some are even beginning to experiment with transferring only one embryo. The ability to culture embryos until Day 5 allows the selection of embryos for transfer from the cohort that have reached the blastocyst stage of development. It is hoped that this advance in IVF treatment will lead to a decrease in the number of embryos that have to be transferred to assure acceptable pregnancy rates.

Embryo transfer

The couple are given a time to come to the unit for embryo replacement. The woman does not need to be fasting since general anaesthesia is not usually required. Depending on the clinical circumstances some women may be asked to come in with a full bladder (Lewin et al., 1997). The couple will first of all have a discussion with the clinician and the embryologist. The treatment results are discussed and the number of embryos for transfer confirmed. If embryos are available for cryopreservation the couple are asked for a signed consent, although this may be clinic specific. Only about one in three couples have enough embryos of good quality to be cryopreserved. Finally, if a video camera is linked to the dissecting microscope, the couple can be shown, on a monitor, the embryos that are to be transferred.

Embryo transfer is usually simple and straightforward. It is not a painful procedure. The woman is positioned appropriately and a vaginal speculum inserted so that the cervix is seen. The cervical os is gently wiped with cotton wool balls moistened with normal saline and then culture medium. At times a pair of vulsellum forceps is applied on the cervix to stabilize it and straighten the angle between the cervical canal and the axis of the uterine cavity thereby making embryo transfer easier. The embryologist picks up all the embryos to be transferred with a thin plastic cannula attached to a syringe and hands over to the clinician (Figure 8.14). The clinician gently inserts the cannula into the uterine cavity through the cervical os and expels the embryos, with a drop of culture medium (Figure 8.15). The cannula is

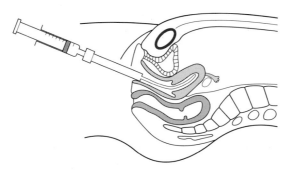

Figure 8.15 Embryo replacement cannula is gently inserted into the uterine cavity and the embryos expelled.

then removed, followed by other instruments and the woman left to lie on the couch for some minutes after which she gets up and goes home. Research has shown that the length of time a woman lies on the couch after the embryo transfer procedure does not affect the subsequent pregnancy rate. It always brings a smile to the otherwise apprehensive patient's face when she is told that 'The embryos will not drop out of the uterus when you stand up!!'. The uterus is usually anteverted or retroverted and in both positions will lie roughly horizontal when the woman is standing. Moreover the anterior and posterior walls of the endometrial cavity usually lie in close apposition to each other thereby sandwiching the embryos between them.

A supply of Cyclogest pessaries adequate for 15 days of use is provided. There does not seem to be much the patient can do to influence the course of events once the embryos have been transferred into the uterine cavity. The most she can be told is to resume her normal activities but avoid doing anything she might later blame herself for doing if she happens not to get pregnant. Some couples may wish to abstain from intercourse for a variable length of time after the transfer. The patient is asked to come back to the hospital for blood to be withdrawn for a pregnancy test if her periods do not start within 12 days after the embryo transfer.

Embryo cryopreservation

Technology is available for cryopreserving embryos. It is however not a perfect science and not all frozen embryos will survive the freezing and thawing process. Furthermore, the pregnancy rate after transfer of frozen-thawed embryos is less than that following transfer of freshly generated embryos. However, the availability of frozen embryos increases the pregnancy potential of each IVF treatment cycle; from one episode of oocyte collection a patient may have two to three episodes of embryo replacement with a cumulative pregnancy rate approaching 60% or more.

Frozen embryos can be stored for a long time but moral complications arise the longer they are left unused. A personal recommendation is that couples should use their stored embryos within three and not more than five years. Options that are available to couples who do not want to use their frozen embryos include donation to other couples who cannot generate embryos of their own. Alternatively the embryos can be used for research into ways of improving the outcome of assisted conception treatments and prevention of the transfer of genetic diseases. Finally, the couple can ask for the embryos to be destroyed. These options can only be exercised after signed consent is obtained from the couple who generated the embryos. Specific details may vary in individual countries.

All couples who have frozen embryos have to contact the IVF unit every year to pay the storage fee for the coming year and sign a form confirming their wish for the embryos to be stored for another year. If they fail to do so they have broken their contract with the IVF unit regarding storage of the embryos. This implies that the IVF unit is legally free to do whatever it believes is justified, which is most commonly the destruction of the embryos. A few years ago, the regulatory body for IVF and similar treatments in the UK ordered the destruction of such 'abandoned' embryos and this was carried out amidst publicity and controversy. The author is not advocating any option within the context of this publication but patients must be made to realize the importance of keeping in touch with the IVF unit if they have embryos that are being stored there.

The fate of the transferred embryos

No one knows exactly what happens to the embryos over the ensuing days following their transfer into the uterine cavity. They may remain at the point of deposition or may drift around the uterine cavity by fluid currents, contractions of the endometrium and/or uterine muscle. The fact that some women have an ectopic pregnancy after IVF treatment implies that some embryos, at least, pass into the fallopian tubes and re-enter the uterine cavity at a later date for implantation. In the natural situation, an ovulated oocyte is fertilized in the fallopian tube within a few hours and then propelled along the fallopian tube to enter the uterine cavity four to five days later and implanting about a day after that. The same might happen to some or all of the embryos that are transferred after IVF. From the time of embryo transfer until implantation is complete the embryos are nourished by nutrient-rich fluid secreted by endometrial cells. The embryo implants by hatching through the zona pellucida and burrowing into the endometrium. It then forms the placenta and starts to develop into a recognizable human being. By the time two weeks have elapsed from the embryo transfer the embryo has already started producing hCG which signals to various organ systems in the mother's

Table 8.7. Success following conventional in vitro fertilization with own oocytes in the UK during 1992

Age of patient	Number of cycles	Clinical pregnancy rates	Livebirth rates
<25	178	16.9	9.6
25–29	2416	22.1	16.5
30–34	6806	19.0	14.6
35–39	6039	15.2	11.4
40–44	2065	8.2	4.5
45 and above	174	3.4	1.7

body that a pregnancy has occurred. hCG is detected in blood or urine by pregnancy tests.

The pregnancy test

The two-week period of waiting for the pregnancy test is a very stressful time. Unfortunately not much can be done about it but psychoprophylaxis can reduce the stress and make the couple better equipped to cope with the period of uncertainty. A sample of the woman's blood is withdrawn for a pregnancy test 14 days from the time of oocyte collection, which normally should be 12 days from the time of embryo transfer. The pregnancy test is rapid and results should be known that same day. The clinician or nurse should phone the couple with the results as soon as they are available that same day. Most times the result is clearly positive or negative. Occasionally, it is equivocal. In this case the actual concentration of hCG is determined in that same blood sample and on another blood sample that is withdrawn 48 hours to one week later.

The success rate of IVF

Success following IVF and other assisted conception treatments can be assessed in a number of ways. The most relevant from the patient's perspective is having a clinical pregnancy and a baby. A clinical pregnancy is a pregnancy that is demonstrated to be viable at the first ultrasound scan that is carried out three weeks after a positive pregnancy test. About 30–40% of women who start each cycle of IVF treatment achieve clinical pregnancies (Meldrum et al., 1998). The success rate depends on several factors many of which are unknown. The known determinants of success include the cause of the infertility, age of the female (Dor et al., 1996), the response to ovarian stimulation, semen quality and the number and appearance of embryos generated and transferred. The effect of age on IVF pregnancy rates is illustrated by the data from the UK which is shown in Table 8.7. Pregnancy rates are lowest in women aged 40 years and above. It is not certain if women who have had children previously or had previous successful IVF treatment cycles have a better chance of falling pregnant with IVF treatment than others who have never been pregnant. Some patients succeed in getting pregnant in the first cycle of treatment while others may require two or more cycles of treatment to do so and some never succeed irrespective of the number of times they have IVF treatment. Some of the pregnancies end in miscarriage (25%) or as ectopic pregnancies (up to 5%) and the proportion of women who will deliver live normal babies will be less; the so-called 'take home baby' rate is about 15%.

This information may be depressing initially but it may not be very different from what happens in nature. About 30% of the so-called fertile population succeed in getting pregnant naturally in the first month of trying. The following month the success rate decreases to say 20–25%. The rate keeps on falling until the sixth month when it is 5%. From then onwards only about 5% of couples who have still not achieved pregnancies succeed in doing so each month. Although the IVF pregnancy rate starts off lower when compared to the 30% rate found in the first month for the fertile population, the rate does not fall appreciably with each cycle of treatment, unlike that obtained in natural conception. When the proportion of couples who succeed in getting pregnant within one year of trying naturally (about 80%) is compared to that found after five cycles of IVF treatment in one year (about 60–70%) it will be seen that there is not much difference in the rates. This way of looking at total conceptions within an extended time frame is called the cumulative pregnancy rate and has changed the way success at IVF treatment is regarded. Conception through IVF and other assisted conception treatments, for a large proportion of couples, is a question of time and the number of attempts. However, everyone, including the medical team, want the treatment to succeed and as soon as possible. This is because of the expensive nature of the treatment, the risk of injury during and after the treatment, associated stress and disruption of the couples' routine and work.

Negative outcome of IVF treatment

Patients in whom the menstrual period commences beforehand do not need to have the pregnancy test since this invariably means that they are not pregnant. If however the bleeding is very scanty and can be described as mere spotting of blood, the test can be performed to clarify issues. Progesterone supplementation is stopped in all women with negative outcome (either negative pregnancy test or commencement of menstrual period) and they are given outpatient clinic appointments. The fact that menstrual periods have not commenced in a female who is on progesterone supplementation after IVF treatment does not necessarily mean that she is pregnant since progesterone can postpone menstrual periods. Menstruation occurs following discontinuation of the pessaries

At the clinic visit the concluded IVF treatment cycle is reviewed and an attempt made to find out why pregnancy did not occur and if any future treatment cycle needs to be modified in any way to improve the chances of successful outcome. Usually, no obvious cause is found for the failed treatment cycle. If embryos were frozen the couple have a choice between having a frozen embryo replacement or accumulating more frozen embryos by having another IVF cycle. The latter option may be considered in a woman whose increasing age is becoming worrisome as it is better to have more oocytes collected sooner than later when the effect of age on oocyte quality becomes more pronounced. The resulting embryos are frozen and can be transferred even when the woman is much older with the expectation of pregnancy rates commensurate with the woman's age when the oocytes were retrieved.

Positive pregnancy test result

Patients who have positive pregnancy test results will continue to insert the Cyclogest pessaries as directed, usually 400 mg twice daily. An ultrasound scan is performed three weeks after the positive pregnancy test. This is to confirm the pregnancy as being intrauterine, check the number and viability of fetuses (Figures 8.16–8.18). If the findings are normal the pessaries are continued for another nine weeks. The patient can gradually decrease the dose of Cyclogest in the last week of use. An example is 200 mg twice daily for four days and 200 mg once a day for three days and then stopping all medication on the eighth day. Alternatively, she can abruptly stop the medication at the stated time without first tailing off the dose in the last week of use.

The timing of ultrasound scans during pregnancy

The age of any pregnancy is conventionally calculated from two weeks before the expected day of fertilization. Thus women who have had successful IVF treatment are regarded as being four weeks pregnant at the time of the pregnancy test which is normally performed two weeks from the day of oocyte collection. It follows that the first ultrasound scan is performed at seven weeks of pregnancy and the use of Cyclogest pessaries is discontinued on completion of the twelfth week of pregnancy. Another ultrasound scan is performed at this time i.e. at 12 weeks. The patient is referred to the antenatal clinic for pregnancy care after the 12 week ultrasound scan. It is advisable to have another scan at 19 and 32 weeks of pregnancy.

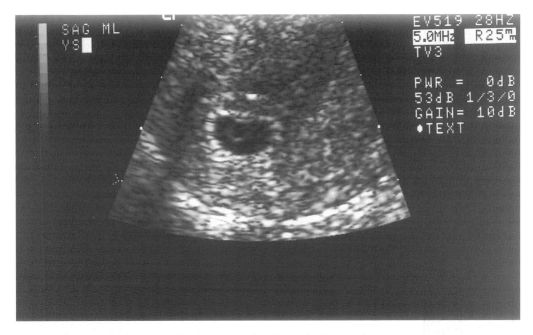

Figure 8.16 An early pregnancy ultrasonogram showing a single gestation sac.

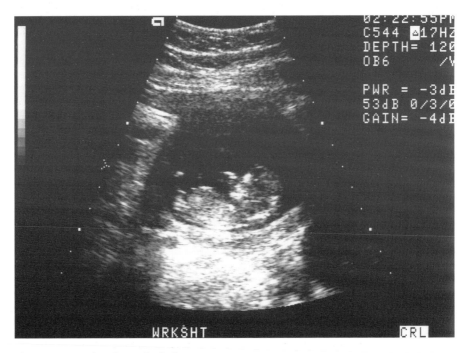

Figure 8.17 Ultrasonogram showing a single fetus.

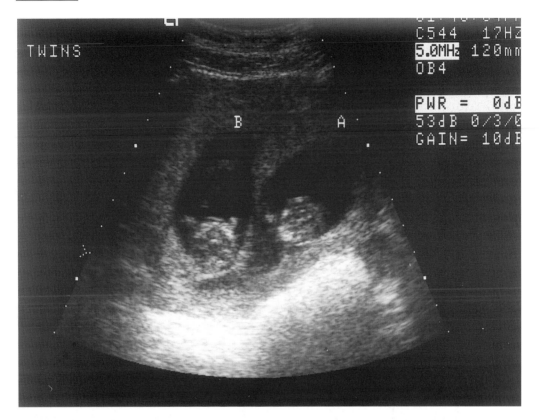

Figure 8.18 Ultrasonogram showing twin pregnancy.

The duration of pregnancy is 40 weeks but women start delivering from two weeks before this time (i.e. 38 weeks) and continue to do so normally until two weeks later (i.e. 42 weeks). While most IVF pregnancies were initially delivered by Caesarean section the indication for this operation nowadays is based more on obstetric factors. However, it is still permissible to perform term elective Caesarean section on social grounds, following successful IVF treatment.

Undesirable aspects of IVF treatment

IVF treatment is expensive and may drain the financial resources of infertile couples. It also imposes a strain on the physical state of the woman and the couple's mental state. The requirement for frequent visits to the IVF unit during the period of treatment disrupts their work routine and special arrangements, including annual leave, may be required. The couple's sex life takes a further beating as the man is asked to produce semen on demand and in unfamiliar environments. The woman is administered several injections some of which may be painful and she has several blood samples withdrawn for different tests. Transvaginal ultrasound scans, although necessary, are still another invasion of the woman's privacy but she puts up with it in the hope that at the end of the day the treatment will be successful.

Minor side-effects of administered drugs and hormones include headaches. Those who sniff GnRHa preparations may have nasal problems arising from irritation of the mucous membranes. There may be allergic reactions to some of the injections. The injections may be painful and cause localized skin reactions including bruising and redness. Some IVF treatment cycles may be cancelled prior to the stage of oocyte collection. The incidence varies but up to 10–15% of treatment cycles can be cancelled. This is usually due to poor response to ovarian stimulation with the number of developing follicles being less than three. Occasionally it may be due to a very excessive response which could become life threatening if hCG is administered and oocyte collection with subsequent embryo transfer is carried out. Premature surging of LH production by the pituitary gland used to be a common cause of cycle cancellation but this is much less common nowadays that GnRHa is being used to suppress pituitary function using the long protocol in a major proportion of patients.

Cramping pain just like 'period time pains' may be felt after oocyte retrieval. This may last for 24–48 hours. There may be slight bleeding from the needle punctures in the vagina following oocyte collection. Occasionally the bleeding may be heavy and require haemostatic sutures on the vaginal wall. A blood vessel may be punctured and bleed inside the pelvis. Bowel loops can also be punctured. The incidence of infection is low; 0.58% has been quoted by some researchers. There is always a chance that none of the oocytes will become fertilized by the sperm. This fertilization failure is mainly due to sperm defects although poor oocyte quality can be implicated at times.

Ovarian response to stimulation may be excessive with the ovaries becoming very enlarged with fluid accumulation in the abdominal cavity (called ascites). In severe cases, there may be fluid accumulation around the heart and lungs (pericardial and pulmonary effusion respectively). Abdominal distension and discomfort are early symptoms and the patient may become very sick and in need of hospital admission and treatment. This is OHSS and is potentially life threatening in the severe variety. The mild type of OHSS (Table 8.8) is present in about 10–25% or more of patients who have IVF treatment. All that is needed is bed rest with increased oral intake of fluid and the use of mild analgesics such as paracetamol. The moderate type of OHSS occurs in less than 5% of patients while the incidence of the severe type is 1–2%.

Patients with moderate or severe OHSS need closer monitoring with ultrasound scans and blood tests (Tables 8.9–8.11). Some of them may require hospital admission and intravenous fluid therapy with colloids and crystalloids (Tables 8.9 and

Table 8.8. Clinical grading of ovarian hyperstimulation syndrome (OHSS)

Grade	Clinical features
Mild	
1	Abdominal distension and discomfort
2	(1) + nausea, vomiting and/or diarrhoea; enlarged ovaries (5–12 cm)
Moderate	
3	Features of mild OHSS + ascites seen on ultrasound scan
Severe	
4	Features of moderate OHSS + ascites diagnosed clinically and/or hydrothorax and breathing difficulties
5	(1) to (4) + haemoconcentration, coagulopathy and diminished renal perfusion and function

Table 8.9. Evaluation of severe ovarian hyperstimulation syndrome

Fluid balance chart
Daily measurement of abdominal girth and body weight
Full blood count (especially haematocrit)
Serum electrolytes, urea and creatinine
Serum albumin and total protein
Liver function tests
Serial abdominal and pelvic ultrasound scans
Clotting studies
Serum and urine osmolarity
Chest X-ray
Central venous pressure
Pregnancy test (two weeks after embryo transfer)

8.10). If ascites is excessive and begins to impact on the respiration, by splinting the diaphragm, the fluid can be removed gradually by needle aspiration (called paracentesis). From experience it is only the ascitic fluid that needs to be tapped; once this is done the patient recovers dramatically, with the urine output increasing.

OHSS is probably the most important complication of assisted conception treatment and all attempts must be made to prevent its development or progression. It may become necessary to withhold the hCG injection and cancel the treatment cycle. Alternatively hCG can be administered and the oocytes collected, fertilized and frozen pending recovery from the OHSS. This is because hCG produced by the embryo following implantation worsens the problem. In future treatment cycles a smaller dose of gonadotrophins is administered to prevent a recurrence of the

Table 8.10. Possible problems in patients with severe ovarian hyperstimulation syndrome

Ovarian enlargement	Ascites
Haemoconcentration	Electrolyte imbalance
Pleural effusion	Hydrothorax
Coagulation defects/thromboembolism	Liver dysfunction
Decreased renal perfusion and oliguria	Torsion of the ovary
Adult respiratory distress syndrome	Cerebrovascular accident

Table 8.11. Principles of treatment in severe ovarian hyperstimulation syndrome

Hospital admission
Correction of electrolyte imbalance with crystalloids
Plasma expansion with colloid solutions such as albumin
Paracentesis
Other supportive therapy
Anticoagulants if indicated

excessive response. There is a suggestion that infusion of hyperoncortic albumin solution (20–25%, w/w) at the time of oocyte retrieval in a woman judged to be at risk of having OHSS may decrease the incidence and severity of the problem (Asch et al., 1993).

The incidence of multiple pregnancy is high because more than one embryo is transferred in order to improve the chances of conception. The incidence of twin pregnancy is 25% and triplets 5% when three embryos are transferred. Quadruplets and higher order gestations are possible because one or more of the three transferred embryos may each divide into two. This is also the reason why a patient who has only one embryo transferred can still have twins and the woman who had two transferred have triplets. The incidence of most complications of pregnancy is increased in multiple pregnancy including miscarriage and premature labour (Table 8.6).

Premature labour is a particular problem especially in triplet and higher order pregnancies. Premature babies may die or spend long periods under intensive care, which is expensive. Many of those who survive have residual problems such as developmental delay and permanently depend on others for sustenance. Some patients may opt for one or more of the multiple fetuses to be reduced (killed with for example lethal injections) early in pregnancy. Although this seems to have doubled the miscarriage rate in some series, those pregnancies that continue have a better outcome since the incidence of premature delivery and other problems decreases. This fetal reduction exposes the couple and medical team to psychological stress and moral dilemmas.

Ectopic pregnancy is more common after IVF treatment than in the normal population but no one knows exactly why this is so. It may relate to the fact that more women who have IVF treatment have tubal problems which predispose them to having ectopic pregnancies. The incidence of ectopic pregnancy after IVF treatment is approximately 3% of all pregnancies. The ultrasound scan that is carried out three weeks after a positive pregnancy test should show a developing pregnancy inside the uterine cavity. If this is not seen, attempts have to be made to find out if there is a tubal ectopic pregnancy. Laparoscopy may be required to exclude ectopic pregnancy in such circumstances. Early detection of an ectopic pregnancy should avoid the dangers that arise when an ectopic pregnancy ruptures. It also widens the scope for more conservative treatment options that will spare the fallopian tube from being excised.

About 25% of IVF pregnancies may miscarry. Initially this incidence appears to be high but studies in the general population indicate a similar miscarriage rate. However, some women, such as those who have polycystic ovary syndrome, have a higher miscarriage rate than others, irrespective of whether they conceive naturally or through IVF treatment.

Some researchers have reported a slight increase in the incidence of ovarian cancer in women who have ovarian stimulation for assisted conception treatment (Harris et al., 1992; Horn-Ross et al., 1992; Whittemore et al., 1992; Whittemore, 1993; Rossing et al., 1994). This is a worrying finding and further research is being carried out to find out if this is actually the case (Balasch & Barri, 1993; Cohen et al., 1993; Venn et al., 1995; Shushan et al., 1996). There is a possibility that this finding is real but the causation of cancer is a very complex ill-understood process and individual susceptibility may influence it. Further research will also provide clues that will help identify those women who are most likely to develop this problem.

Welfare of IVF babies

Babies delivered as a result of IVF treatment and other assisted conception treatments do not seem to have a congenital malformation rate that is greater than that of the normal population (less than 5%). Behaviourally they are similar to other children, although they are loved and pampered a little more than usual! Their fathers have been found to show more interest in their daily care more than fathers of babies who were conceived naturally. There is no evidence at present to show that their development is different from that of other children and young adults. The first IVF baby, who was born in 1978, is now in her twenties.

Counselling and psychoprophylaxis

Infertility can evoke profound psychological reactions in some couples and may alter their perception of life. One of the notable features is that of feeling intensely helpless and alone. Assisted conception treatments are complex and stressful. There is need for support, and counselling facilities are provided. Couples are ideally seen by the counsellor prior to commencing treatment, during the treatment and afterwards especially if the treatment fails. The role of counselling in assisted conception treatments cannot be overemphasized and couples are strongly advised to avail themselves of that service.

Please, tell them to keep in touch!

It is important for couples to keep in touch with the IVF unit and notify relevant staff of the outcome of their pregnancy. This will help in keeping accurate records which have formed the basis for most research that is carried out in this area. Such research aims at improving further the results of treatment. In some countries it is required by law that units should notify the regulatory agency of treatment outcome. The medical team know all their patients by name and remain interested in their welfare long after they have completed their treatment. Although it is not happy news they would still like to know if their patients miscarry, have ectopic pregnancies or any other undesirable outcome. They are ecstatic when they hear of a recent delivery. They are even happier when pictures of babies start arriving and they eventually visit the unit with their parents. It is not just the babies; pictures of toddlers and young children adorn the walls of many units and they act as testimony of the work that is being carried out to assist infertile couples obtain one of life's greatest gifts.

Conclusion

Conventional IVF treatment has assumed a prominent role in the management of infertile couples and is continually under evaluation to improve further the success of the treatment. It is important that patients are carefully selected but early rather than late referral will ensure that their chances of having successful treatment are optimized.

BIBLIOGRAPHY

Asch, R. H., Ivery, E., Goldsman, M. et al. (1993). The use of intravenous albumin in patients at high risk for severe ovarian hyperstimulation syndrome. *Fertility and Sterility* 8, 1015–20.

Balasch, J. & Barri, P. N. (1993). Follicular stimulation and ovarian cancer? *Human Reproduction* **8**, 990–6.

Ben-Chetrit, A., Senoz, S. & Greenblatt, E. M. (1997). In vitro fertilization programmed for weekday-only oocyte harvest: analysis of outcome based on actual retrieval day. *Journal of Assisted Reproduction and Genetics* **14**, 26–31.

Cohen, J., Forman, R., Harlap, S. et al. (1993). IFFS expert group report on the Whittemore study related to the risk of ovarian cancer associated with the use of infertility agents. *Human Reproduction* **8**, 996–9.

Devreker, F., Emiliani, S., Revelard, P. et al. (1999). Comparison of two elective transfer policies of two embryos to reduce multiple pregnancies without impairing pregnancy rates. *Human Reproduction* **14**, 83–9.

Dor, J., Seidman, D. S. & Ben-Shlomo, I. (1996). Cumulative pregnancy rate following in vitro-fertilization: the significance of age and infertility aetiology. *Human Reproduction* **11**, 425–8.

Edwards, R. G., Lobo, R. & Bouchard, P. (1996). Time to revolutionize ovarian stimulation. (Editorial.) *Human Reproduction* **11**, 917–19.

Egbase, P. E., Al-Sharhan, M., Al-Mutawa, M. et al. (1996). Mimicking the high levels of activity of a large in-vitro fertilization unit leads to early success at the commencement of an in-vitro fertilization and embryo transfer programme. *Human Reproduction* **11**, 2127–9.

Engmann, L., Maconochie, N., Bekir, J. & Tan, S. L. (1999). Progestogen therapy during pituitary desensitization with gonadotropin-releasing hormone agonist prevents functional ovarian cyst formation: a prospective, randomized study. *American Journal of Obstetrics and Gynecology* **1181**, 576–82.

Gardner, D. K., Schoolraft, W. B., Wagley, L. et al. (1998a). A prospective randomized trial of blastocyst culture and transfer in in-vitro fertilization. *Human Reproduction* **13**, 3434–40.

Gardner, D. K., Vella, P., Lane, M. et al. (1998b). Culture and transfer of human blastocysts increases implantation rates and reduces the need for multiple embryo transfers. *Fertility and Sterility* **69**, 84–8.

Harris, R., Whittemore, A. S., Intyre, J. & the Collaborative Ovarian Cancer Group (1992). Characteristics relating to ovarian cancer risk: collaborative analysis of 12 US case-control studies. III. Epithelial tumors of low malignant potential in white women. *American Journal of Epidemiology* **136**, 1204–11.

Horn-Ross, P. L., Whittemore, A. S., Intyre, J. & the Collaborative Ovarian Cancer Group (1992). Characteristics relating to ovarian cancer risk: collaborative analysis of 12 US case-control studies. VI. Nonepithelial cancers among adults. *Epidemiology* **3**, 490–5.

Lewin, A., Schenker, J. G., Avrech, O. et al. (1997). The role of uterine straightening by passive bladder distension before embryo transfer in IVF cycles. *Journal of Assisted Reproduction and Genetics* **14**, 32–4.

Lin, Y., Kahn, J. A. & Hillensjo, T. (1999). Is there a difference in the function of granulosa-luteal cells in patients undergoing in-vitro fertilization either with gonadotrophin-releasing hormone agonist or gonadotrophin-releasing hormone antagonist? *Human Reproduction* **14**, 885–8.

Matson, P. L., Browne, J., Deakin, R. & Bellinge, B. (1999). The transfer of two embryos instead of three to reduce the risk of multiple pregnancy: a retrospective analysis. *Journal of Assisted Reproduction and Genetics* **16**, 1–5.

Meldrum, D. R., Silverberg, K. M., Bustillo, M. & Stokes, L. (1998). Success rate with repeated cycles of in vitro fertilization-embryo transfer. *Fertility and Sterility* **69**, 1005–9.

Meniru, G. I. & Craft, I. L. (1997). Utilization of retrieved oocytes as an index of the efficiency of superovulation strategies for in-vitro fertilization treatment. *Human Reproduction* **12**, 2129–32.

Pados, G., Talatzis, B. C., Bontis, J. et al. (1995). Evaluation of different ovarian stimulation protocols for in vitro fertilization. *Gynecological Endocrinology* **9**, 103–12.

Pouly, J. L., Bassil, S., Frydman, R. et al. (1996). Luteal support after in-vitro fertilization: Crinone 8%, a sustained release vaginal progesterone gel, versus Utrogestan, an oral micronized progesterone. *Human Reproduction* **11**, 2085–9.

Rongieres-Bertrand, C., Oliveness, F., Righini, C. et al. (1999). Revival of the natural cycles in in-vitro fertilization with the use of a new gonadotrophin-releasing hormone antagonist (Cetrorelix): a pilot study with minimal stimulation. *Human Reproduction* **14**, 683–8.

Rossing, M. A., Daling, J. R., Weiss, N. S. et al. (1994). Ovarian tumors in a cohort of infertile women. *New England Journal of Medicine* **331**, 771–6.

Shushan, A., Paltiel, O., Iscovich, J. et al. (1996). Human menopausal gonadotropin and the risk of epithelial ovarian cancer. *Fertility and Sterility* **65**, 13–18.

Steptoe, P. C. & Edwards, R. G. (1978). Birth after the reimplantation of a human embryo. *Lancet* **2**, 336. (Letter.)

Tsirigotis, M., Hutchon, S., Yazdani, N. & Craft, I. (1995.) The value of oestradiol estimations in controlled ovarian hyperstimulation cycles. *Human Reproduction* **10**, 972–3. (Letter.)

Venn, A., Watson, L., Lumley, J. et al. (1995). Breast and ovarian cancer incidence after infertility and *in vitro* fertilization. *Lancet* **346**, 995–1000.

Weissman, A., Meriano, J., Ward, S. et al. (1999). Intracytoplasmic sperm injection after follicle stimulation with highly purified human follicle stimulating hormone compared with human menopausal gonadotropin. *Journal of Assisted Reproduction and Genetics* **16**, 63–8.

Whittemore, A. S. (1993). Fertility drugs and the risk of ovarian cancer. *Human Reproduction* **8**, 999–1000.

Whittemore, A. S., Harris, R., Intyre, J. & the Collaborative Ovarian Cancer Group (1992). Characteristics relating to ovarian cancer risk: collaborative analysis of twelve US case-control studies. II. invasive epithelial ovarian cancer in white women. *American Journal of Epidemiology* **136**, 1184–203.

9

Intracytoplasmic sperm injection

Introduction

The management of male factor infertility has until recently been very problematic, inefficient and not very rewarding. This derives partially from the fact that the cause of depressed semen parameters may be unknown in a large proportion of cases. Even where a cause is found the subnormal testicular function or the genital tract lesion is invariably irreversible; many medical and surgical treatment methods have failed to provide a cure for male factor problems that translate into improved pregnancy rates. With the introduction of assisted conception technology into clinical practice, attempts have been made to discover more efficient methods of treating infertile couples with male factor problems (Table 9.1).

Artificial insemination with sperm from the partner has been found useful in some couples with mild to moderate depression of semen parameters; intrauterine insemination with washed partner sperm following mild superovulation is associated with an improved pregnancy rate provided that the total motile sperm count after sperm washing is greater than one million (Ombelet et al., 1995; Campana et al., 1996). Following early successes in women with tubal infertility, conventional in vitro fertilization (IVF) was evaluated for use in male factor infertility cases. Again, while it was of some use in some cases, there was a tendency towards failed fertilization or poor fertilization rates when the sperm abnormality was moderate or severe. Variants of conventional IVF have been used in an attempt to overcome the lowered fertilization potential of sperm from men with some degree of depression of the normal sperm parameters. These include HIC-IVF (high insemination concentration IVF) and μIVF (microdrop-IVF). In the first method the concentration of sperm in the insemination culture dish is increased. This has been found to be successful in some cases while not being helpful in others. Moreover it is possible that the higher concentration of metabolic products arising from the large number of sperm in the culture medium may exert toxic effects on the oocytes and resulting embryos. Reducing the volume of culture medium in the insemination dish (μIVF) will have the same affect of concentrating the few available sperm after

Table 9.1. Assisted conception treatment methods used to overcome male factor infertility

Artificial insemination with partner sperm (intrauterine insemination)
Conventional in vitro fertilization
High insemination concentration in vitro fertilization
Microdrop in vitro fertilization
Sperm motility stimulants
Zona drilling
Partial zona dissection
Subzonal insemination
Intracytoplasmic sperm injection

sperm preparation. The cumulus cells surrounding the oocytes are removed, prior to transferring them to the microdroplet of sperm suspension. This is to remove the extra impediment presented by the cumulus mass to sperm ingress and allow the accommodation of several oocytes within the microdroplet. The assisted conception treatment method of gamete intrafallopian transfer (GIFT, discussed more fully in Chapter 11) has been used in patients with male factor problems with a similarly inconsistent trend in pregnancy rates being observed especially when there is moderate to severe abnormality of semen parameters.

Another area of endeavour has been the use of stimulants to improve sperm motility and the potential for fertilization. Such stimulants include pentoxifylline, caffeine, 2-deoxyadenosine and follicular fluid. Although some workers achieved improved fertilization rates when prepared sperm were pre-incubated in culture medium containing any of these compounds, other researchers did not have similar results; moreover there still remained a core group of patients whose semen parameters were so subnormal that even the use of sperm motility stimulants was not an option for them.

The microassisted fertilization technique also has been tried (Figure 9.1). The aim of this technique is to bypass the oocyte's natural barriers to fertilization. In zona drilling (ZD) a small hole is made in the zona pellucida with acid Tyrode's solution or acid phosphate-buffered saline solution thereby making it easier for sperm to reach the perivitelline space hopefully to fuse with the oolemma. Alternatively, the hole may be drilled with a fine needle. Partial zona dissection (PZD) involves creating a slit in the zona pellucida with a fine glass needle or micro-blade while subzonal insemination (SUZI) involves the injection of a few motile sperm, (usually 5–8), into the perivitelline space with the expectation that a sperm will fuse with the oolemma and fertilize the oocyte. These microassisted fertilization methods were of limited efficacy and associated pregnancy rates continued to be low. Furthermore, there was a higher risk of more than one sperm fertilizing

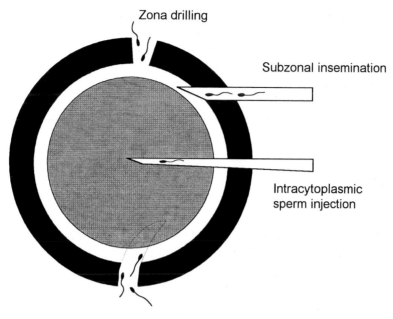

Zona drilling

Subzonal insemination

Intracytoplasmic
sperm injection

Partial zona dissection

Figure 9.1   Schematic representation of microassisted fertilization techniques.

each oocyte (polyspermic fertilization). The most recent microassisted fertilization method is called intracytoplasmic sperm injection (ICSI) and involves the injection of a single sperm into the cytoplasm of the oocyte. Reports began appearing in scientific journals in 1992 of consistently successful treatment outcomes following clinical application of ICSI. The reports were initially made by the group of workers at the Dutch-speaking Brussels Free University led by Professor Andre Van Steirteghem. ICSI is now widely available in a large number of assisted conception units internationally and has revolutionized the management of male factor infertility. ICSI is associated with fertilization and pregnancy rates similar to those found following conventional IVF in patients who do not have male factor problems. The following is a simplified account of how ICSI is performed. It is meant to be informative rather than technically exhaustive; specific technical details are available in standard texts for laboratory staff and interested clinicians. Supervised practical training is required for certification of competence in this area.

Indications

ICSI is indicated in any infertile couple in whom there is a significant chance of failed or very poor fertilization following treatment with conventional IVF (Table 9.2). Such couples include those with a previous history of a similar event. While it

Table 9.2. Indications for intracytoplasmic sperm injection

Previous failed fertilization

Marked depression of semen parameters:

 sperm concentration < 5 million/ml

 progressive motility < 10%

 normal morphology < 4%

 total motile sperm count after sperm preparation < 1 million

Borderline semen parameters

Specific patients groups:

 retrograde ejaculation

 impotence necessitating electroejaculation

 severe seminal antisperm antibody problem

 frozen poor quality sperm (e.g. from testicular cancer patients)

Sperm retrieved from patients with initial diagnosis of azoospermia

In vitro matured oocytes

Poor quality donor sperm

is common to state that such a failure has to be repeated at least once before offering the couple ICSI it is not clear how well this dictum is followed in assisted conception units. This is because the emotional and financial involvement of assisted conception treatment demands that couples achieve pregnancy in as few treatment cycles as possible. Following failed fertilization at conventional IVF treatment all aspects of the treatment are evaluated to determine the cause. This will include microscopic examination of the oocytes, assessing their quality and the presence of sperm binding to the zona pellucida. Finally, a diagnostic ICSI is carried out on the unfertilized oocytes to find out if they will become fertilized. At the end of the review it may be possible to identify patients in whom a repeat conventional IVF treatment is bound to fail and those with equivocal or normal results. The latter group of patients may have another trial at conventional IVF but some units will carry out this type of insemination on only half of the retrieved oocytes while ICSI is performed on the other half as a safeguard. If the fertilization rate is satisfactory in the group of oocytes exposed to conventional IVF it means that this should remain the method of choice if further assisted conception treatment is required in future.

A group of patients who will benefit from having ICSI at the outset rather than conventional IVF are those who have a marked depression of their semen parameters. This includes patients with moderate to severe oligo-, astheno-, and/or teratozoospermia. Again, pressure may be brought to bear upon the clinician to resort more readily to ICSI, even in men with borderline semen analysis results. As yet, there is still no test that can accurately predict all patients who will have failed fertilization from conventional IVF as a result of a defect in the sperm. It may be prudent to offer ICSI if the concentration of sperm in the ejaculate is less than 5 million/ml or the progressive motility is less than 10%. Some authorities will not consider ICSI unless the total motile sperm count after sperm preparation is less than one million. Still others adopt very strict criteria for grading the morphology of each sperm and establishing cut-off points (such as 4%) below which ICSI is chosen to assure normal fertilization rates. Invariably, the decision to use ICSI as the insemination method of choice in some patients will depend on a combination of factors that denote a poor prognosis for fertilization using conventional IVF. As was seen in earlier chapters (especially Chapters 4 and 6) no cause will be found in a substantial proportion of men with subnormal semen parameters. These and other patient groups with more recognizable aetiologies (retrograde ejaculation, impotence leading to the use of electroejaculation, high concentration of seminal antisperm antibodies and testicular/other cancer patients) have benefited immensely from the availability of ICSI. Studies have shown that couples where the man has borderline semen analysis results fare much better with ICSI than with conventional IVF. A simple rule to follow whenever there is doubt about the most appropriate insemination method to apply is to split the retrieved oocytes into two groups; one group is inseminated by conventional IVF and the other by ICSI. If fertilization in the IVF group is satisfactory, any future treatments should be by conventional IVF and vice versa.

Patients with azoospermia are increasingly being offered ICSI as it is possible to recover sperm, by surgical means, from the genital tract or testes of these men if the azoospermia is obstructive in origin (Meniru et al., 1998). Even in patients with non-obstructive azoospermia, it may be possible to recover sperm from the ejaculate in up to 35% of cases, after long periods of painstaking search of the pellet obtained by centrifuging the semen sample at high speeds for up to 30 minutes (Ron-El et al., 1997). A similar proportion of patients with non-obstructive azoospermia will have sperm recovered from testicular tissue. The quality of sperm retrieved from these patients is poor but the powerful effect of ICSI is such that reasonable fertilization rates and pregnancies result despite this. Surgical sperm retrieval has been adequately covered in Chapter 10.

ICSI is used in achieving fertilization of in vitro matured oocytes irrespective of how normal the man's semen parameters are. Prolonged in vitro culture of immature oocytes is currently being evaluated as another means of providing mature oocytes for assisted conception treatment. The oocytes are either aspirated from immature ovarian follicles or obtained from pieces of tissue that have been removed surgically from the ovary. Ovarian biopsy and freezing is becoming more common in females who have to undergo anticancer treatment with chemotherapy or radiotherapy. Animal experiments have shown that such tissue can be thawed and cultured successfully to produce mature oocytes. However, prolonged in vitro culture may cause hardening of the zona pellucida thereby making sperm penetration unpredictable or impossible. ICSI can be performed successfully on such oocytes and some human pregnancies have already been reported in the scientific literature (Young et al., 1998).

Meniru et al. (1997) have reported on the use of ICSI with donor sperm. There has been a fall in the number of males who come forward to donate sperm for infertile couples in some parts of the world such as UK and Europe. In other places, cultural or religious reasons may make it difficult to recruit prospective donors. This has led to sperm banks accepting donors with relatively poor semen parameters especially if from an ethnic group from which it is difficult to recruit donors. When confronted with a poor donor sperm sample most assisted conception units will usually use a better sample from another donor. In so doing sperm is prepared for use in artificial insemination or conventional IVF. However, in cases where alternative donor sperm samples are unavailable, HIC-IVF and μIVF can be attempted, but our experience showed that this did not improve the fertilization results – there was still an unacceptably high failed fertilization rate. This led to a change in policy at the London Gynaecology and Fertility Centre to the use of ICSI whenever the donor sperm sample was poor and there were no alternative samples of better quality.

Provision of sperm for ICSI

A broad spectrum of male factor problems and patients are found during ICSI treatment. Their peculiar problems and requirements have to be appreciated for an efficient trouble free ICSI procedure to be carried out. Some patients may have poor but stable semen parameters; these patients will invariably produce semen with roughly the same parameters each time a sample is required. They are judged to be at low risk of having unexpected azoospermia or impotence on the day of oocyte retrieval. In such instances, they are asked to produce a fresh semen sample on the morning of oocyte collection for use during ICSI. Some others may have been diagnosed as having deteriorating semen samples and would be required to have some sperm frozen prior to the day of oocyte collection. This will also include men who have had their semen samples frozen prior to chemotherapy or radiotherapy for testicular or other malignancies. Some patients may have episodic impotence or find it impossible to masturbate on demand especially in the hospital premises. It is prudent for these men to produce semen samples at home and at their convenience, and bring the samples to the unit for cryopreservation before their partners commence superovulation induction. There are still some other groups of patients

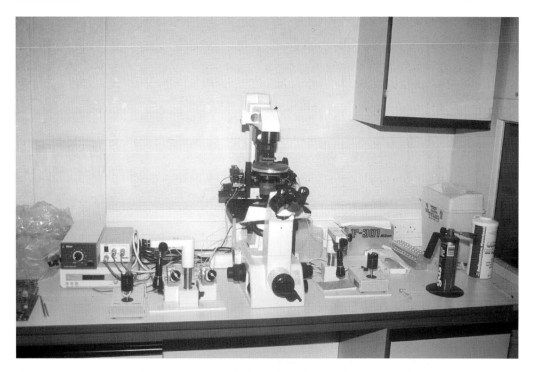

Figure 9.2   A Nikon Diaphot microscope with Narishige micromanipulating equipment and microinjectors.

in whom it will be most convenient to have their sperm frozen before the morning of oocyte retrieval such as men requiring electroejaculation and surgical sperm retrieval. The technology of sperm freezing is sufficiently reliable, and sperm survival after freezing and thawing is predictable provided a test thaw analysis is carried out on one of the frozen ampoules of sperm after a day or two of cryostorage. In some instances the frozen sperm is kept as backup in case the man is not able to produce a sample on the day of oocyte retrieval or the quality of the fresh semen sample is worse than that of the frozen sample.

Instrumentation

The use of the right type of equipment is probably the single most important determinant of success at ICSI. At the heart of the equipment set up is an inverted phase-contrast microscope such as the Nikon Diaphot 200 or 300 (Nikon Corporation, Tokyo, Japan) that is equipped with a Hoffman modulation contrast system (Modulation Optics Inc., Greenvale, USA) (Figure 9.2). The Nomarski system is an alternative contrast system and it allows colour photography. The stage of the microscope is heated keeping the temperature between 37 °C and 38 °C so that the

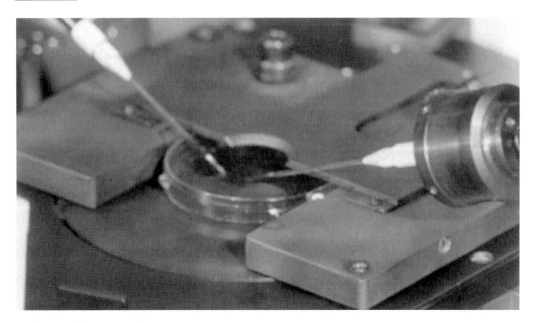

Figure 9.3   Close up view of a microscope stage showing the electrically heated metal plate on which the dish containing the gametes is placed.

gametes are maintained at body temperature while outside the incubator (Figure 9.3). Micromanipulating equipment is mounted on the microscope for use during the ICSI procedure. A holder for the needle is mounted on each side. Each needle holder is linked by Teflon tube to a microinjector. There are micromanipulators for coarse movements of the needles and others for fine movement. The needles can be made to move rapidly or slowly in various directions such as up, down, forwards, backwards, to the left, to the right and in a circular manner along the horizontal axis. There is now a wide array of equipment of differing complexity. Micromanipulators made by Research Instruments Ltd., (Penryn, Cornwall, UK) (Figure 9.4) and Narishige Co. Ltd., (Tokyo, Japan) (Figure 9.2) are both of high standards and there are still other brands in the market. Finely pulled glass needles are mounted on the micromanipulators using the needle holders. The needle that is mounted usually on the left side is blunt ended and used for holding the oocyte to allow the injection of sperm using the sharp needle that is mounted on the right needle holder. Connected to these needles are microinjectors which provide very finely controlled suction and ejection forces (Figure 9.5a,b). Initially, most units fabricated their injection needles using equipment similar to those shown on Figures 9.6(a–d) but this is labour intensive and best left to dedicated manufacturing concerns which hopefully should produce high quality and standardized needles for ICSI. Many such companies are now in operation. The needles are purchased already cleaned and sterilized ready for use. They are discarded after

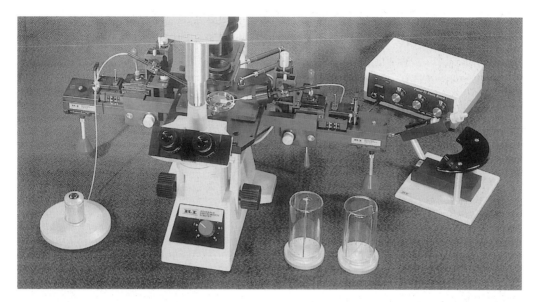

Figure 9.4   Micromanipulators and microinjectors from Research Instruments Ltd., UK, mounted on an Olympus CK2–Tri microscope.

(a)
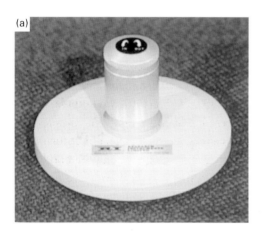

(b)
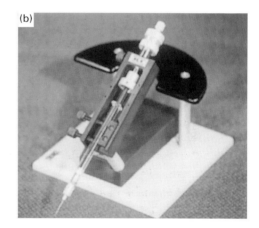

Figure 9.5   Microinjectors from Research Instruments Ltd., UK: (a) SAS syringe: injection and aspiration is by air displacement; (b) MSHD micrometer syringe: oil filled and generates hydraulic pressure for injection and aspiration.

being used for ICSI of a patient's oocytes. Usually one injection needle is adequate for the injection of all the oocytes of one patient. However, it may be changed if it becomes blunt or is clogged by debris. The micromanipulation equipment is set up on a vibration-free surface in a room that is free of human traffic or in a quiet part of the IVF laboratory. A few minutes before ICSI is started, fresh needles are mounted on the holders and positioned appropriately.

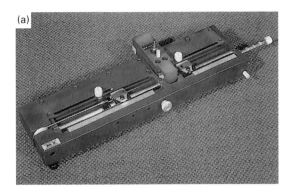

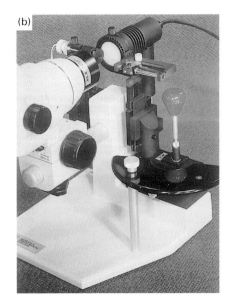

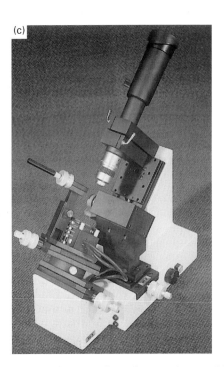

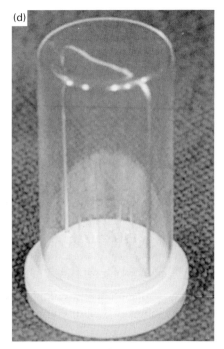

Figure 9.6 Microinjection needle making equipment from Research Instruments Ltd., UK: (a) electrically heated micropipette puller; (b) microforge used for cutting and thermally polishing the needle tip, reduction of the needle lumen diameter at the tip and introduction of the required needle bend; (c) turbo-microbeveller for grinding the sperm injection needle tip; (d) pipette storage container.

Superovulation and oocyte retrieval

Multiple follicular development is stimulated with individualized dose regimens of follicle stimulating hormone preparations and/or human menopausal gonadotrophin usually using the long protocol of pituitary desensitization as described in Chapter 8. Transvaginal oocyte aspiration, under intravenous sedation, is carried out 36 hours after the administration of an ovulatory injection of human chorionic gonadotrophin. The aspirated oocytes are incubated in culture medium for one to three hours before removing the cumulus cells.

Sperm preparation

The processing of sperm samples is carried out using different methods depending on the quality of the sample and observed sperm motility. Density gradient centrifugation initially was carried out with Percoll but other media such as PureSperm that have been developed specifically for human use are now used instead. An aliquot of the sperm sample is gently layered over a discontinuous gradient of 1.5 ml of 45% PureSperm and 1.5 ml of 90% PureSperm (Figure 9.7) and centrifuged at $500 \times g$ for 10 minutes. The pellet is resuspended in fresh gamete culture medium and centrifuged at $500 \times g$ for 10 minutes. The washing step is repeated with another aliquot of fresh culture medium. The pellet is then resuspended in fresh culture medium and the sperm concentration adjusted to about 1 million/ml.

The use of gradient density centrifugation may not be appropriate for all sperm samples because recovery of motile sperm can be unpredictable in poor sperm samples and often less than desired. Simple washing and swim-up (Figure 9.8) or washing alone may be better for such samples. Sperm washing is performed by adding about 4–5 ml of culture medium to 1–3 ml of the sperm sample in a centrifuge tube. The sample is centrifuged at $500 \times g$ for 10 minutes. The pellet is resuspended in 5 ml of culture medium and spun again at $500 \times g$ for 10 minutes. Following this the supernatant is carefully removed to leave just about 1 ml of clear culture medium above the pellet and the tube placed for 30 minutes to one hour in an incubator maintained at 37 °C in a 5% CO_2-in-humidified-air mixture. At the end of this incubation period the tube is carefully removed from the incubator and the fluid lying above the sperm pellet, which usually contains sperm that have swum up from the pellet, is gently removed and transferred to a fresh tube. If motile sperm is not recovered from the fluid above the pellet, the pellet is resuspended in culture medium and used for ICSI as described in one of the following sections. The concentration of sperm, following successful sperm preparation, is adjusted to

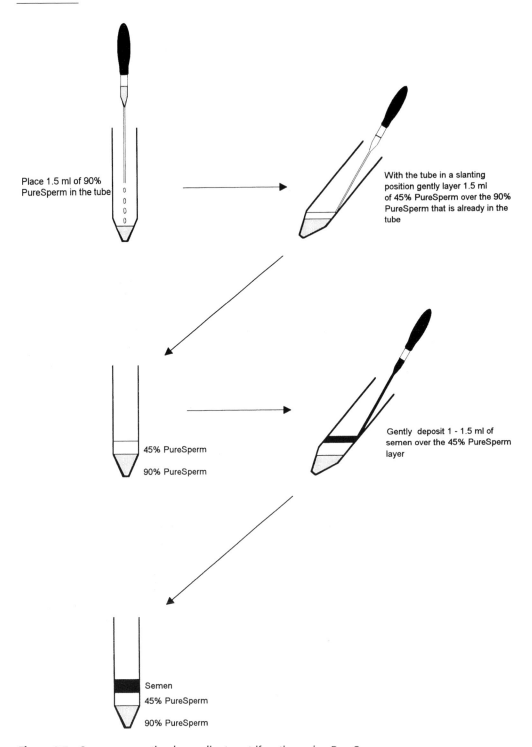

Place 1.5 ml of 90% PureSperm in the tube

With the tube in a slanting position gently layer 1.5 ml of 45% PureSperm over the 90% PureSperm that is already in the tube

45% PureSperm

90% PureSperm

Gently deposit 1 - 1.5 ml of semen over the 45% PureSperm layer

Semen

45% PureSperm

90% PureSperm

Figure 9.7   Sperm preparation by gradient centrifugation using PureSperm.

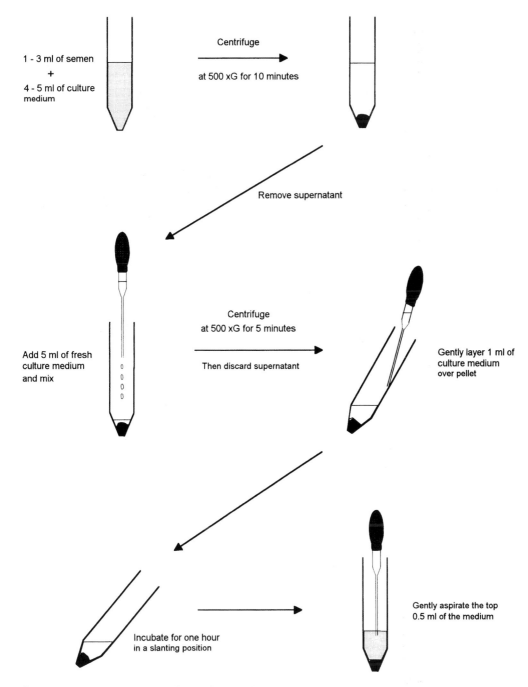

1 - 3 ml of semen
+
4 - 5 ml of culture medium

Centrifuge
at 500 xG for 10 minutes

Remove supernatant

Add 5 ml of fresh culture medium and mix

Centrifuge
at 500 xG for 5 minutes

Then discard supernatant

Gently layer 1 ml of culture medium over pellet

Incubate for one hour in a slanting position

Gently aspirate the top 0.5 ml of the medium

Figure 9.8   Sperm preparation by washing and swim-up.

(a)

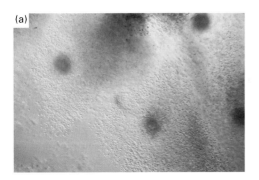

(b)

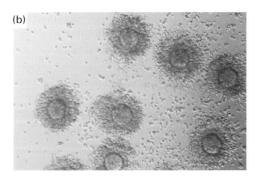

(c)

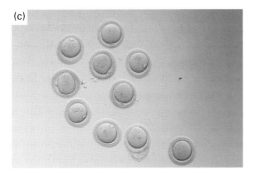

Figure 9.9 Photomicrograph showing stages during removal of surrounding cumulus cells from retrieved oocytes: (a) the oocyte-cumulus complexes (OCC) have just been transferred into the hyaluronidase solution; (b) the OCC have now been transferred into fresh culture medium and some of the cumulus cells have already been removed; (c) the cumulus cells have been completely removed from the oocytes allowing visualization of the first polar body in metaphase II oocytes.

about 1 million/ml by adding measured volumes of culture medium to the sperm suspension. The tube of prepared sperm suspension is returned to the incubator until required for ICSI.

Removal of cumulus cells

Prior to the ICSI procedure the retrieved oocytes are denuded of their surrounding cumulus cells (Figure 9.9). This is accomplished by transferring the oocytes into a culture dish containing hyaluronidase solution (60–80 IU/ml). Hyaluronidase is an enzyme that digests a component of the connective tissue elements that hold cells together. After about one minute the oocytes are removed and transferred into a dish containing fresh culture medium. The oocytes are then drawn in and out of finely drawn sterile glass pipettes with an inner diameter of approximately 150–200 µm. Following complete removal of the cumulus cells the oocytes are washed in fresh culture medium and carefully examined under high magnification (×200). Only oocytes that have reached metaphase of the second meiotic division are selected; this is the stage of development in which the oocyte is seen to have

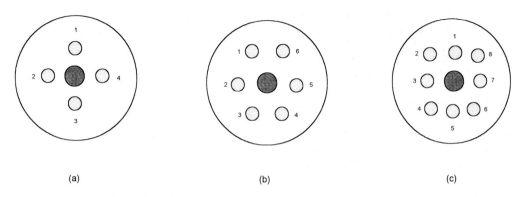

(a)　　　　　　　　　　　(b)　　　　　　　　　　　(c)

Figure 9.10 Different arrangements for the placement of culture medium and polyvinylpyrrolidone (PVP) droplets in the dish that will be used for intracytoplasmic sperm injection: (a) four droplets of culture medium surrounding the PVP droplet; (b) six droplets of culture medium surrounding the PVP droplet; (c) eight droplets of culture medium surrounding the PVP droplet.

extruded the first polar body into the perivitelline space. The oocytes are subsequently cultured in fresh medium until the time of injection.

Preparation of the dish for injection

A special electrostatically coated dish is used for holding the gametes for ICSI. A 10 μl microdroplet of polyvinylpyrrolidone (PVP) is placed at the centre of the dish. About 1 μl of the prepared sperm suspension is placed at the middle of this PVP droplet. PVP is a viscous fluid and is used to slow down motile sperm making it easy for the sperm to be caught with the injection pipette prior to ICSI. Four to eight other droplets are placed round the PVP droplet as shown in Figure 9.10. These are 5 μl droplets of culture medium in which the oocytes will be placed for ICSI. About 4–5 ml of liquid paraffin is gently poured into the dish to cover these droplets to reduce evaporation from their surfaces during the time of ICSI. The dish is then returned to the incubator for about 30 minutes before transferring the oocytes into the culture droplets ready for ICSI.

ICSI

The ICSI dish is positioned on the microscope stage such that the PVP droplet is in view. The injection pipette is lowered into the droplet and a small amount of PVP aspirated (Figure 9.11). The needle is next used in scoring the tail of one of the slowly moving sperm (Figure 9.12) and then aspirating the sperm, tail first, into the pipette.

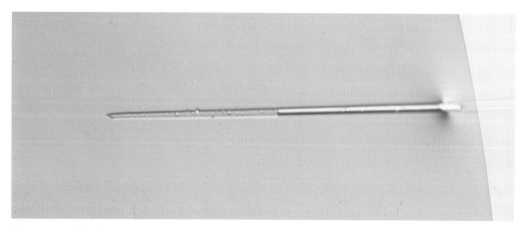

Figure 9.11 Injection pipette just lowered into polyvinylpyrrolidone droplet.

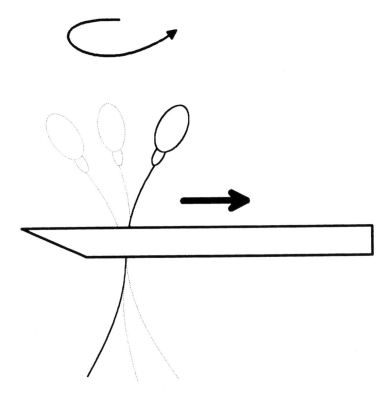

Figure 9.12 Diagram showing scoring of the sperm tail with the injection pipette prior to sperm pick-up. The injection needle is rested on the tail of a motile sperm which it then presses against the floor of the dish while it (the injection needle) is moved outwards. When performed correctly the sperm can be seen to rotate during the manoeuvre and the tail will become kinked. This controlled damage to the sperm tail is thought to release factors that are important for fertilization events in the injected oocytes.

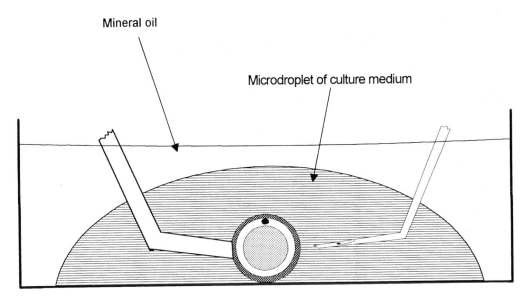

Mineral oil

Microdroplet of culture medium

Figure 9.13 Diagrammatic representation of an oocyte being held with the holding pipette with the polar body at the 12 o'clock position.

The injection pipette is raised above the dish and the dish manoeuvred around such that the first oocyte-containing droplet is brought into view. The oocyte holding pipette is lowered into this droplet followed by the injection pipette. The holding pipette is gently brought to the side of the oocyte and slight suction pressure applied such that the oocyte is held firmly with the polar body at the 12 or 6 o'clock position (Figure 9.13). The injection pipette enters the oocyte with a quick movement from the side opposite to that of the holding pipette. There is usually some tenting of the oolemma but it gives way with more inward movement of the needle. Following entry of the needle tip into the cytoplasm a slight suction movement is made with the microinjector resulting in a small portion of the cytoplasm flowing backwards into the injection needle. This step is necessary to confirm that the needle has indeed pierced the oolemma. There is also some evidence to suggest that such agitation of the cytoplasm is required for activation of the oocyte leading to commencement of changes that will bring about fertilization. The aspirated cytoplasm is then expelled back into the oocyte followed closely by the sperm. The injection needle is withdrawn from the oocyte. The negative pressure in the holding pipette is released thereby releasing the oocyte. The needles are removed from the droplet and raised above the dish which is moved around to bring the central PVP droplet into view again. The sequence of sperm pick up and oocyte injection is repeated until all oocytes are injected and this is illustrated in Figures 9.14 to 9.16. The injected oocytes are washed with fresh culture medium and returned to the incubator in a fresh culture dish.

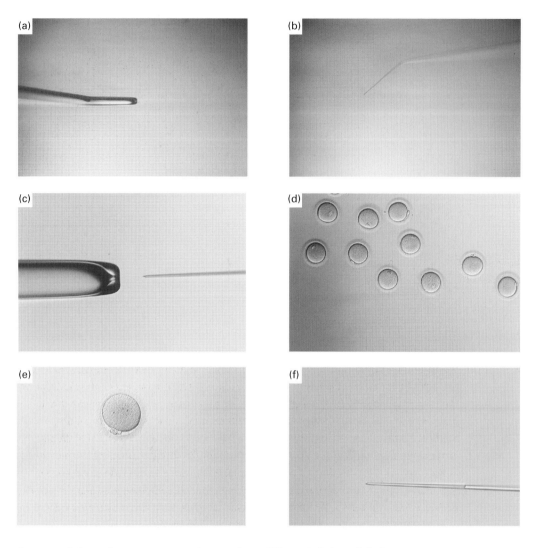

Sperm pick-up from processed samples still containing debris

When the processed sperm sample is still contaminated by cellular debris and immotile sperm, either of two techniques can be used to avoid the injection of these contaminants along with the sperm during ICSI. If the motile sperm demonstrates progressive motility, 2 μl of the sample is carefully placed at the centre of a 10 μl droplet of PVP. Drops of culture medium are placed around the PVP droplet to hold the oocytes during injection. These drops are overlaid with equilibrated liquid paraffin. Following 30 minutes of incubation motile sperm would often have moved to the edge of the PVP droplet. Such sperm are easily picked up with the injection pipette for ICSI. When significant progressive motility is absent in a sperm sample three droplets of the sample are placed proximal to the PVP droplet

(g)

(h)
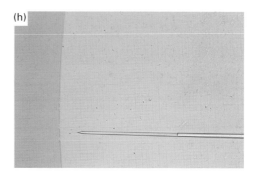

(i)
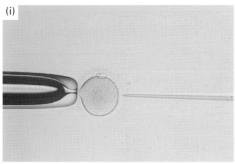

Figure 9.14 Stages during intracytoplasmic sperm injection: (a) the holding pipette is mounted on the left side of the micromanipulator; (b) the injection pipette is mounted on the right side of the micromanipulator; (c) the alignment of both pipettes is checked; (d) metaphase II oocytes ready for injection; (e) one of the oocytes is moved to a droplet of culture medium ready for injection; (f) the injection pipette is lowered into the central droplet containing slowly moving sperm; (g) the dish is moved around to bring the edge of the droplet in view; (h) the injection pipette is used to aspirate sperm found at the edge of the droplet; and, (i) the oocyte is held with the left mounted pipette such that the polar body is either at the 12 or 6 o'clock position and the injection pipette may be used in manipulating the oocyte around to achieve the desired positioning.

while four droplets of culture medium are placed distally for the oocytes (Figure 9.17). The injection pipette is first placed in the PVP droplet to aspirate a small volume of PVP so as to improve pipette control during sperm pick up from the sperm suspension droplet. Furthermore the PVP fluid column makes it possible to eject the sperm and cellular debris completely into the central PVP droplet without blowing air bubbles. After picking up the sperm from the sperm suspension, it is washed free of any debris in the PVP droplet, the tail scored with the injection pipette followed by sperm aspiration and ICSI. Scoring of the sperm tail is necessary because this releases chemical compounds called cytosolic factors that will aid the activation of the injected oocyte.

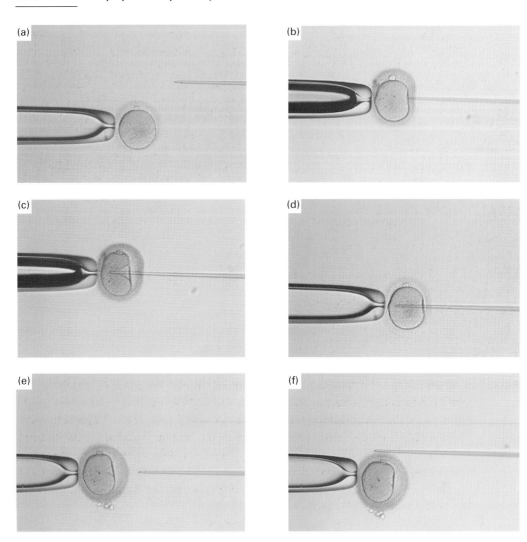

Fertilization, embryo culture and transfer

The injected oocytes are inspected 12–18 hours later for signs of fertilization. Some may be seen to have been damaged during the injection. They appear dull and brownish giving a ground glass appearance (Figure 9.18). Normally fertilized oocytes have two pronuclei and are transferred into fresh culture dishes and replaced in the incubator. Abnormal fertilization patterns include eggs showing one pronucleus, three pronuclei or more; these are discarded. The subsequent culture of normally fertilized eggs and other aspects of the treatment are similar to that of conventional IVF. A maximum of three cleaving embryos is replaced in the uterus approximately 48–72 hours after oocyte retrieval. Any remaining good quality embryos are cryopreserved.

(g)

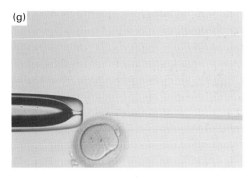

(h)

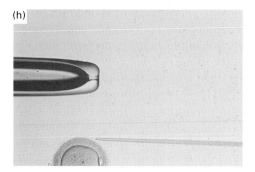

(i)

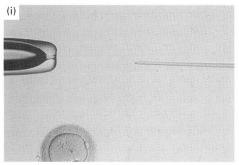

Figure 9.15 Stages during intracytoplasmic sperm injection:(a) the oocyte is held with the left mounted pipette while the right mounted pipette has been used to pick up a sperm from the central droplet ready for injection; (b) the injection pipette is pressed against the side of the oocyte; (c) the pipette pierces the zona pellucida of the oocyte and presses against the oolemma causing its tenting; (d) the pipette pierces the oolemma and the sperm is deposited in the cytoplasm of the oocyte; (e) the injection pipette is withdrawn from the oocyte; and (f–i) the suction pressure in the holding pipette is released and the injection needle used to push the oocyte away.

The luteal phase is supplemented with natural progesterone pessaries. Patients have a serum β-hCG pregnancy test 12 days after embryo transfer. Those with positive test results continue using progesterone pessaries until 8–12 weeks of pregnancy, as discussed in Chapter 8. Transvaginal ultrasound scans are performed three weeks after the positive pregnancy test to confirm clinical pregnancy and determine whether there is a multiple pregnancy.

ICSI data

Several thousand ICSI treatment cycles have now been carried out internationally with generally similar trends being observed in terms of the results. Perhaps it is appropriate that data on outcome to be presented here should be from the pioneer

(a)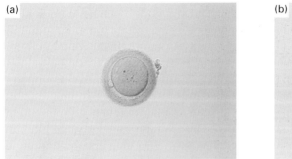

(b)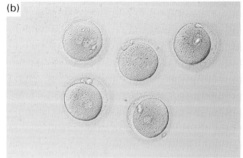

Figure 9.16 Stages during intracytoplasmic sperm injection: (a) appearance of the oocyte a few minutes after intracytoplasmic sperm injection; and (b) normally fertilized oocytes each with two pronuclei.

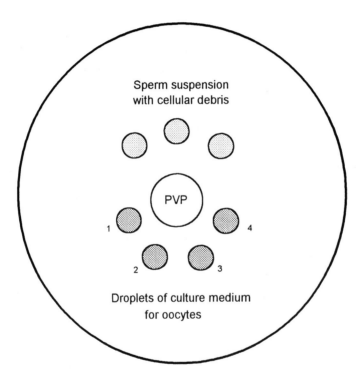

Figure 9.17 Arrangement of droplets for sperm pick-up and intracytoplasmic sperm injection when the prepared sperm sample still contains a significant amount of cellular debris.

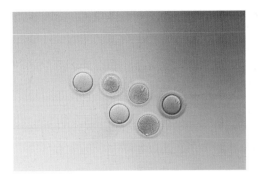

Figure 9.18. Three damaged oocytes following intracytoplasmic sperm injection compared with three oocytes that survived the injection. Damaged (lysed) oocytes have a dull brownish appearance.

institution. A summary of their experience was presented at the third Bourn Hall (Cambridge, UK) reunion meeting (Van Steirteghem et al., 1996) (Table 9.3). Most of the patients included in that report (2572 cycles or 91.2%) had ICSI with ejaculated sperm while epididymal sperm was utilized in 128 cycles (4.5%) and testicular sperm used in 120 cycles (4.3%). The average normal (two pronuclei) fertilization rate was 62.4% but it was significantly higher in patients who had ICSI with ejaculated sperm when compared to the rate obtained when epididymal and testicular sperm were used. There is always a chance of an oocyte being damaged during ICSI. A poor injection technique obviously will lead to damage of oocytes just as with the use of large calibre or blunt injection needles. The oocyte quality may be a factor as well (Loutradis et al., 1999). It has been observed, for example, that oocyte damage is more common when the oolemma does not offer any resistance to the piercing action of the injection needle. It seems that some degree of tenting of the oolemma will occur in normal oocytes during insertion of the injection needle. The loss of oolemma elasticity may be a marker of poor oocyte quality. As a general rule a 10% damage rate should be expected following ICSI. This damage rate may be reduced in future when the aetiology of oocyte damage during ICSI becomes better understood and avoidable. The cleavage rate of the normally fertilized eggs is commonly 90% and above. The subsequent development of the embryos appears to be controlled more by factors of maternal origin such as age than by the male factor problem. Positive pregnancy test results will be obtained in 35% or more of patients who have embryo transfer. The clinical pregnancy and delivery rates will be slightly lower than this but usually 20–25% and above. At times one gets the impression that ICSI has a slightly better pregnancy rate than conventional IVF but the issue of relative efficacy of these procedures will be addressed better in future. The author's ICSI results from the laboratory phase of

Table 9.3. Results of assisted conception treatment with intracytoplasmic sperm injection

	Brussels Free University*		Author's experience		
	Number	%	Number	%	Denominator for %
ICSI Cycles	2820	n/a	135	n/a	n/a
Metaphase II eggs injected	29415	n/a	1266	n/a	n/a
2 pn	18364	62.4	925	73.0	Injected metaphase II eggs
0 pn	5679	19.3	111	8.8	same
1 pn	991	3.4	87	6.9	same
3 pn	1194	4.1	23	1.8	same
Oocytes damaged by the injection procedure	3187	10.8	98	7.7	same
Fertilized eggs that cleaved into embryos	?	?	835	90.3	Normally fertilized (2 pn) eggs
Patients having embryo transfer	2608	92.5	134	99.3	ICSI Cycles
Transferred embryos	6744	36.7	370	40.0	Normally fertilized (2 pn) eggs
Frozen embryos	5239	28.5	320	34.6	Normally fertilized (2 pn) eggs
Positive pregnancy test result	964	36.9	54	40.3	Patients having embryo transfer

Notes: 2pn: 2 pronuclei; 0pn: no pronucleus; 1pn: 1 pronucleus; 3pn: 3 pronuclei.
Source: Van Steirteghem et al. (1996)

his fellowship training in Reproductive Medicine are also shown in Table 9.3. The source of sperm for the ICSI procedures was ejaculated semen in 119 couples (88%), PESA (percutaneous epididymal sperm aspiration) in 12 couples (9%) and TESA (testicular sperm aspiration) in 4 couples (3%).

Welfare of ICSI babies

Since ICSI bypasses most of the anatomical and physiological sperm screening mechanisms normally presented by both the female genital tract and oocyte it follows that there will be disquiet regarding the welfare of the fetus and resulting child. This is especially true in patients where the sperm quality is very poor forcing a decision to inject sperm that is barely moving or has an abnormal shape. A point to bear in mind is that the sperm is designed for motility carrying a copy of a man's genetic material through various obstacles and into the oocyte. However, a sperm with defective motility or morphology may not necessarily be carrying defective chromosomes in its nucleus. On the other hand some male factor problems may have a genetic origin. Well-known examples include congenital bilateral absence of the vas deferens (CBAVD) in patients who are carriers of cystic fibrosis mutant genes and immotile sperm in patients with Kartagener's syndrome. Other examples exist and recent findings have shown that some males with subnormal semen parameters in the absence of a specific phenotype may have microdeletions in their Y chromosome. In these instances, ICSI does not necessarily cause a new genetic problem but makes it possible for the couple to have children, some or all of whom may inherit their parents' genetic disorders. Preconception genetic evaluation and counselling of these couples, and probably all couples who have ICSI treatment, should be carried out. Pre-implantation genetic diagnosis, chorionic villus sampling and/or amniocentesis should be offered to all patients. If a couple who have an obvious inheritable problem insist on being treated with ICSI what should be the clinician's response? The consequences of agreeing are obvious but refusal to provide the treatment places the clinician at risk of being accused of denying the couple their fundamental right to procreate or 'trying to play God' by deciding who should and who should not have children.

Another area of concern is whether there is any aspect of the ICSI treatment which in itself introduces a disorder or predisposes the resulting child to having peculiar health problems at birth, infancy, adolescence, adulthood or old age, or passing on mutations, for example, to their descendants. Unfortunately, at present this is an area where a 100% assurance cannot be provided to couples. It is only with close and prolonged monitoring of individuals who are conceived as a result of ICSI that some of these concerns can be fully addressed. The Brussels team have led the way in this area by counselling couples to have pre-natal genetic diagnosis and then follow-up checks from birth. Their most current reviews (Bonduelle et al., 1996, 1998) have not documented any increase in the chromosomal abnormality rate or the incidence of major malformations in babies resulting from ICSI when compared to rates found in the general population. Of course this information needs to be updated periodically, as more babies are born and the children get older. Similar trends have been documented in other studies (Wennerholm et al., 1996; Loft et al., 1999)

Spermatid injection

A careful microscopic examination of semen produced by men with non-obstructive azoospermia may reveal spermatids in about 70% of cases. It has been shown that injection of these spermatids may result in the fertilization of about

43% of the injected oocytes. A much larger proportion of the normally fertilized eggs then divide to form embryos. Some human pregnancies have now been reported globally (Fishel et al., 1995; Bernabeu et al., 1998; Sofikitis et al., 1998). The spermatids are separated from other cellular components of semen by using protocols similar to the one shown in Figure 9.19. There are two broad varieties of spermatids that are recognized in semen, the round and elongated spermatids. Injection of round spermatids into oocytes is called ROSI (round spermatid injection) while injection of the elongated spermatid is called ELSI (elongated spermatid injection). The fertilization rate following intracytoplasmic injection of elongating or elongated spermatids is significantly higher than that obtained with injection of round spermatids. A report has documented a fertilization rate of 71% with ELSI compared to that of 25.6% with ROSI (Kahraman et al., 1998). Although initial pregnancy rates have been lower than that of ICSI using fully formed sperm (found in the testis, epididymis or ejaculate) (Gordts et al., 1998; Ghazzawi et al., 1999) there is hope that further refinements of the technique will result in higher pregnancy rates. At present spermatid injection represents the last option for men with secretory azoospermia in whom mature sperm cannot be recovered from the ejaculate, genital tract or testis. Some workers feel that spermatid injection should be performed instead of surgical sperm retrieval in patients with secretory azoospermia. It is also possible to find free-lying spermatids in testicular tissue samples.

Conclusion

ICSI has forever changed the management of male factor infertility. While not signalling the end of attempts at full clinical and laboratory evaluation, and medical or surgical treatment of male factor problems, there is now assurance that if those treatments fail or are not appropriate to the case in question, an effective assisted conception treatment option is available. It should also decrease the application of ineffective medical and surgical remedies. Enthusiasm in applying ICSI should however be tempered because there is no long-term data on the welfare of progeny and it will be a long time before this becomes available, certainly not in our lifetime. It is therefore important that every practitioner should apply this treatment with the greatest degree of responsibility and good faith. The only defence we presently have for the rapid application of the new assisted reproductive technologies in clinical practice is that we do not have more conservative time-tested treatment options that are equally or nearly as effective. This is, however, not the only area where difficult ethical and moral decisions have to be made in medical care. It is also not the only situation where self-proclaimed guardians of the human race have tried to dictate to others while shying away from a candid appraisal of their individual motives and the relationship to their life experience or lack of. Advances in

Centrifuge liquefied semen at 1200 xg for 10 minutes

Resuspend pellet in 1 ml of culture medium

Place on top of a discontinuous gradient density centrifugation medium

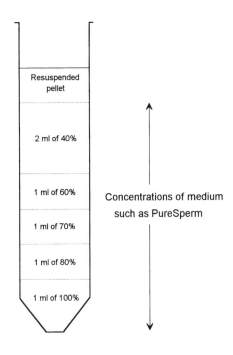

Centrifuge at 330 x *g* for 20 minutes

Carefully aspirate the 70% layer and transfer to a fresh tube

Add 10 ml of culture medium, mix and centrifuge at 600 x *g* for 10 minutes

Remove supernatant and resuspend pellet in another 10 ml of culture medium

Centrifuge at 600 x *g* for 10 minutes

Resuspend pellet in 0.5 ml of culture medium and place in incubator until required

Figure 9.19 Scheme showing stages during the extraction of spermatids from a semen sample (Adapted from Tesarik & Mendoza, 1996).

medicine and science have always outpaced contemporary societal views and norms and are most likely to be viewed, at least initially, with scepticism and suspicion especially by those who are not in immediate need of the innovation. A common-sense approach and seeking the assistance of an ethics committee may provide humane solutions in difficult situations.

BIBLIOGRAPHY

Bernabeu, R., Cremades, N., Takahashi, K. & Sousa, M. (1998). Successful pregnancy after spermatid injection. *Human Reproduction* **13**, 1898–900.

Bonduelle, M., Legein, J., Buysse, A. et al. (1996). Prospective follow-up study of 423 children born after intracytoplasmic sperm injection. *Human Reproduction* **11**, 1558–64.

Bonduelle, M., Wilikens, A., Buysse, A. et al. (1998). A follow-up study of children born after intracytoplasmic sperm injection (ICSI) with epididymal and testicular spermatozoa and after replacement of cryopreserved embryos obtained after ICSI. *Human Reproduction* **13**, 196–207.

Campana, A., Sakkas, D., Stalberg, A. et al. (1996). Intrauterine insemination: evaluation of the results according to the woman's age, sperm quality, total sperm count per insemination and life table analysis. *Human Reproduction* **11**, 732–6.

Cummins, J. M. & Jequier, A. M. (1995). Concerns and recommendations for intracytoplasmic sperm injection (ICSI) treatment. *Human Reproduction* **10** (Suppl. 1), 138–43.

Edwards, R. G., Tarin, J. J., Dean, N. et al. (1994). Are spermatid injections into human oocytes now mandatory? (Opinion.) *Human Reproduction* **9**, 2217–19.

Fishel, S., Green, S., Bishop, M. et al. (1995). Pregnancy after intracytoplasmic injection of spermatid. *Lancet* **345**, 1641–2.

Fishel, S., Aslam, I. & Tesarik, J. (1996). Spermatid conception: a stage too early, or a time too soon? (Opinion.) *Human Reproduction* **11**, 1371–5.

Ghazzawi, I. M., Alhasani, S., Taher, M. & Souso, S. (1999). Reproductive capacity of round spermatids compared with mature spermatozoa in a population of azoospermic men. *Human Reproduction* **14**, 736–40.

Gordts, S., Rombauts, L., Roziers, P. et al. (1998). Intracytoplasmic sperm injection in the treatment of male subfertility. *European Journal of Obstetrics and Gynecology and Reproductive Biology* **81**, 207–11.

Kahraman, S., Polat, G., Samli, M. et al. (1998). Multiple pregnancies obtained by testicular spermatid injection in combination with intracytoplasmic sperm injection. *Human Reproduction* **13**, 104–10.

Loft, A., Peterson, K., Erb, K. et al. (1999). A Danish national cohort of 730 infants born after intracytoplasmic sperm injection (ICSI) 1994–1997. *Human Reproduction* **14**, 2143–8.

Loutradis, D., Drakakis, P., Kalliandis, K. et al. (1999). Oocyte morphology correlates with embryo quality and pregnancy rate after intracytoplasmic sperm injection. *Fertility and Sterility* **72**, 240–4.

Mendoza, C. & Tesarik, J. (1996). The occurence and identification of round spermatids in the ejaculate of men with non-obstructive azoospermia. *Fertility and Sterility* **66**, 826–9.

Meniru, G. I., Podsiadly, B. T. & Craft, I. L. (1997). Intracytoplasmic injection of donor spermatozoa. *Human Reproduction* **12**, 1367.

Meniru, G. I., Gorgy, A., Batha, S. et al. (1998). Studies of percutaneous epididymal sperm aspiration (PESA) and intracytoplasmic sperm injection. *Human Reproduction Update* **4**, 57–71.

Nagy, Z. P., Liu, J., Joris, H. et al. (1995). The influence of the site of sperm deposition and mode of oolemma breakage at intracytoplasmic sperm injection on fertilization and embryo development rates. *Human Reproduction* **10**, 3171–7.

Ombelet, W., Cox, A., Jansen, M. et al. (1995). Artificial insemination (AIH). Artificial insemination 2: using the husband's sperm. In *Diagnosis and Therapy of Male Factor in Assisted Reproduction*, ed. A. A. Acosta & T. F. Kruger, pp. 397–410. Carnforth: The Parthenon Publishing Group.

Palermo, G. D., Alikani, M., Bertoli, M. et al. (1996). Oolemma characteristics in relation to survival and fertilization patterns of oocytes treated by intracytoplasmic sperm injection. *Human Reproduction* **11**, 172–6.

Palermo, G. D., Cohen, J. & Rosenwaks, Z. (1996). Intracytoplasmic sperm injection: a powerful tool to overcome fertilization failure. *Fertility and Sterility* **65**, 899–908.

Palermo, G. D., Schlegel, P. N., Colombero, L. T. et al. (1996). Aggressive sperm immobilization prior to intracytoplasmic sperm injection with immature spermatozoa improves fertilization and pregnancy rates. *Human Reproduction* **11**, 1023–9.

Ron-El, R., Strasseburger, D., Friedler, S. et al. (1997). Extended sperm preparation: an alternative to testicular sperm extraction in non-obstructive azoospermia. *Human Reproduction* **12**, 1222–6.

Sofikitis, N. V., Yamamoto, Y., Miyagawa, I. et al. (1998). Ooplasmic injection of elongating spermatids for the treatment of non-obstructive azoospermia. *Human Reproduction* **13**, 709–14.

Tesarik, J. & Mendoza, C. (1996). Spermatid injection into human oocytes. I. Laboratory techniques and special features of zygote development. *Human Reproduction* **11**, 772–9.

Tesarik, J., Rolet, F., Brami, C. et al. (1996). Spermatid injection into human oocytes. II. Clinical application in the treatment of infertility due to non-obstructive azoospermia. *Human Reproduction* **11**, 780–3.

Vanderzwalmen, P., Bertin, G., Lejeune, B. et al. (1996). Two essential steps for a successful intracytoplasmic sperm injection: injection of immobilized spermatozoa after rupture of the oolemma. *Human Reproduction* **11**, 540–7.

Van Steirteghem, A. C., Nagy, P., Joris, H. et al. (1996). The development of intracytoplasmic sperm injection. *Human Reproduction* **11** (Suppl. 1), 59–72.

Wennerholm, U. B., Bergh, C., Hamberger, L. et al. (1996). Obstetric and perinatal outcome of pregnancies following intracytoplasmic sperm injection. *Human Reproduction* **11**, 1113–19.

Young, E., Kenny, A., Puigdomenech, E. et al. (1998). Triplet pregnancy after intracytoplasmic sperm injection of cryopreserved oocytes: case report. *Fertility and Sterility* **70**, 360–1.

10

Surgical sperm retrieval

Introduction

The introduction of intracytoplasmic sperm injection (ICSI) into routine clinical practice (Van Steirteghem et al., 1996) has had a dramatic effect on the management of severe male factor infertility. This is because only a few spermatozoa are needed to ensure the fertilization of retrieved oocytes, using this technique. If, for example, 10 mature oocytes are retrieved from a woman's ovaries following superovulation, it means that only 10 live spermatozoa will be required; one spermatozoon will be injected into each oocyte. This is unlike conventional in vitro fertilization (IVF) in which several thousand spermatozoa are added to the culture dish to ensure that one spermatozoon is able to fertilize each oocyte. Pregnancy rates following ICSI are comparable with rates obtained following conventional IVF in couples who do not have male factor problems (Aboulghar et al., 1996). This powerful effect of ICSI has consequently led to reconsideration of the management of certain male factor problems which were previously regarded as being incompatible with genetic parentage; the patients had invariably required the use of donor spermatozoa for insemination of their partners or the couple had adopted children or led a child-free existence. A number of operative techniques have now been developed for the recovery of spermatozoa from the testes and other parts of the male genital tract (Table 10.1). The quantity and quality of recovered spermatozoa are invariably poor but as results have shown this does not have a major effect on success rates following ICSI provided live spermatozoa can be extracted from the sample and used for the injection. This chapter will deal with some of the more commonly utilized surgical sperm retrieval procedures after a brief review of the indications.

Indications for surgical sperm retrieval

Irremediable obstructive azoospermia was and still remains the main indication for surgical sperm recovery (Temple-Smith et al., 1985; Tournaye et al., 1997) (Table 10.2). Congenital bilateral absence of the vas deferens (CBAVD) is the most

Table 10.1. Surgical sperm retrieval methods

Technique	Acronym
Percutaneous epididymal sperm aspiration	PESA
Microepididymal sperm aspiration	MESA
Testicular sperm aspiration	TESA
Testicular sperm extraction	TESE
Vas deferens sperm aspiration	–
Rete testis aspiration	–
Spermatocoele aspiration	–
Sperm reservoir	–

Table 10.2. Indications for surgical sperm retrieval in 151 patients who had percutaneous epididymal sperm aspiration

Male factor problem	Number	Percentage
Obstructive lesions		
Congenital bilateral absence of the vas deferens	55	36.4
Failed reversal of vasectomy	57	37.7
Unreversed vasectomy	6	4.0
Blockage of the vas deferens following genital tract infection	6	4.0
Ejaculatory duct obstruction	3	2.0
Blockage of the vas deferens in Kartageners syndrome	1	0.7
Young's syndrome	2	1.3
Non-obstructive lesions		
Anejaculation	4	2.6
Impotence	3	2.0
Secretory azoospermia	7	4.6
Severe oligoasthenoteratozoospermia	2	1.3
Incomplete spermatogenic arrest	5	3.3

Notes: Meniru et al. (1997b).

common cause of obstructive azoospermia in men with primary infertility. There is an association between CBAVD and cystic fibrosis. Up to 50% or more of men with CBAVD have been shown to be carriers of cystic fibrosis transmembrane conductance regulator gene mutations (Chillon et al., 1995; Mercier et al., 1995; Schlegel et al., 1995; Shtainer & Nagler, 1995). It is therefore important that both the man and the woman are offered counselling support and genetic testing for cystic fibrosis carrier status. If both partners have the mutation there is a real chance that their offspring will have the disease. If the woman is not a carrier, the most their child can be is a carrier but in the male offspring there will be an increased chance of having CBAVD.

The incidence of failed vasectomy reversal, as a cause of obstructive azoospermia in those desirous of pregnancy, mirrors the extent of utilization of vasectomy for permanent birth control in the population. It is higher in areas where the uptake of vasectomy is high and vice versa (Meniru et al., 1997b). Surgical sperm retrieval can also be performed on some patients with unreversed vasectomy. This includes: (1) men in whom an excessive length of the vas deferens was removed at the time of the initial vasectomy operation thereby making it impossible to rejoin the cut ends of the vas deferens; or (2) the interval between the vasectomy and request for reversal is deemed by the surgeon to be too long for the reversal operation to succeed (Meniru et al., 1996); and (3) men who do not want vasectomy reversal but want surgical sperm retrieval for ICSI treatment of their wives. Obstruction of the vas deferens can be due to inflammatory damage following prolonged or improperly treated genital tract infection. Obstructive azoospermia has been diagnosed in a patient with the Kartageners syndrome (Meniru et al., 1998) although the syndrome normally consists of situs inversus, chronic sinusitis and bronchiectasis in association with defects of sperm tails and cilia of the respiratory tract. In Young's syndrome, there is obstructive azoospermia but testicular production of spermatozoa is normal. Patients with the Young's syndrome also have chronic sinusitis and pulmonary infections. Other indications for surgical sperm retrieval are shown in Table 10.2. Essentially, spermatozoa may be recovered from the genital tract or testes in cases where, for one reason or the other, spermatozoa cannot be found in the ejaculate or the man does not ejaculate at all. Quite surprisingly, spermatozoa can be recovered from the testes of some men who have been clinically diagnosed as having secretory azoospermia (Devroey et al., 1995; Tournaye et al., 1999).

Microepididymal sperm aspiration (MESA)

The first pregnancy to result from MESA was reported by Temple-Smith and colleagues in 1985; retrieved spermatozoa had been used for conventional IVF then. Nowadays, virtually all patients have ICSI when surgically retrieved spermatozoa have to be used for insemination of the retrieved oocytes. MESA involves making an incision through the scrotal skin to reach the contents of the scrotum. The tunica vaginalis (covering layer) is incised to expose the testis and epididymis. The covering of the epididymis is then incised, under the guidance of an operating microscope or magnifying loupes, to expose the underlying epididymal tubules (Figure 10.1). A very small incision is then made into one of the epididymal tubules, a tiny needle or hollow glass rod is passed into the lumen of the epididymal tubule and used in aspirating any fluid found in that segment of the epididymis (Figure 10.2).

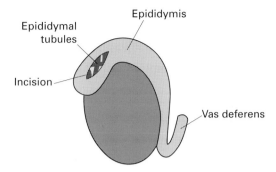

Figure 10.1 An incision is made in the tunica of the epididymis to expose the underlying epididymal tubules.

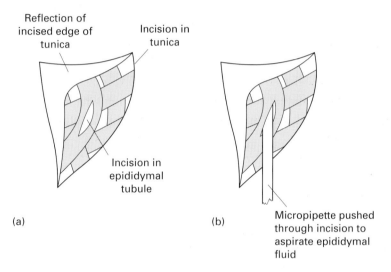

Figure 10.2 Magnified views of: (a) an incised epididymal tubule; and (b) a fine needle or hollow glass rod being inserted into the lumen of the tubule to aspirate fluid.

Alternatively, instead of incising the epididymal tubule a very small glass needle is used in traversing the wall of the tubule and aspirating fluid from the lumen of the tubule (Figure 10.3). The aspirated fluid is flushed out of the needle and tubing with a small amount of culture medium and is collected into a small sterile test tube. A drop of this fluid is examined immediately under the microscope to determine if there are spermatozoa and whether they are motile. This procedure is repeated on several tubules until an adequate number of spermatozoa is deemed to have been recovered. Some of the recovered spermatozoa are immediately used for ICSI treatment while the rest are frozen for possible use in future treatment cycles.

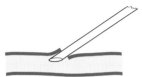

Figure 10.3 A sharp glass pipette is used to puncture an epididymal tubule during microepididymal sperm aspiration.

MESA is successful in 55% or more of cases (Silber et al., 1995; Madgar et al., 1996). Higher retrieval rates are generally achieved by experienced practitioners. The success rate is, however, reduced if there are adhesions and fibrosis in the region of the epididymis. Such scarring can result from exploratory operations which were used to assess the nature of the blockage or attempts at reversing a vasectomy. Scar tissue limits visual access to the epididymal tubules. Scarring can also result from a previous MESA procedure. MESA depends on visualization of the epididymal tubules with expensive microsurgical equipment and highly trained uroandrologists are usually required to perform the operation. The problem with this state of affairs is that it places MESA beyond the reach of many assisted conception units. The patient may be required to stay overnight after the operation or is treated on a day-case basis. Some surgeons have modified the operation such that only a small scrotal incision is required and the testes do not have to be delivered outside the scrotum.

Complications are possible after MESA and include bleeding, infection and haematoma formation in the short-term. In the long-term, there is a tendency towards adhesions and fibrosis at the site of operation. This usually involves the epididymis and makes repeat operations difficult or impossible. General anaesthesia is required for the operation although local anaesthesia can also be used. Post-operative pain is significant and the patient may need to take some days off work to recover after the procedure. Patients are not likely to agree to a repeat operation if this becomes necessary in future.

Exponents of MESA believe that only one MESA procedure is required to supply spermatozoa for use in several ICSI treatment cycles. The recovered spermatozoa are frozen in several plastic ampoules or straws and thawed as required. This is the reason why they believe that the uncertain outcome of repeat MESA should not be taken as a serious point against continuing to use that procedure, irrespective of the fact that there are now alternative and less invasive retrieval procedures.

Percutaneous epididymal sperm aspiration (PESA)

The shortcomings of the MESA procedure have led to the development of a less invasive alternative in the form of PESA (Shrivastav et al., 1994; Craft & Shrivastav,

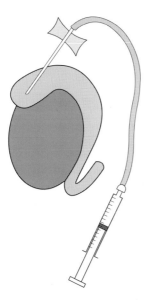

Figure 10.4 Schematic representation of the positioning of a butterfly needle in the epididymis during percutaneous epididymal sperm aspiration.

1994; Craft et al., 1995). This procedure is based on the principles of fine needle aspiration biopsy; negative suction on a needle that is inserted into a defined part of the body often results in the aspiration of cell-laden fluid, in the case of the epididymis, spermatozoa. PESA is performed by stabilizing the epididymis between the index finger, thumb and forefinger while cupping the testis with the palm of the left hand, and pushing the tip of a 21G butterfly needle through the stretched scrotal skin and into the substance of the epididymis (Figure 10.4). Negative pressure is created in the system by fully drawing back the plunger of an attached 20 ml syringe. The tip of the needle is gently moved inwards and outwards within the epididymis until columns of slightly opalescent fluid are seen to be rising in the needle tubing. The vacuum is maintained by applying a pair of artery forceps on the tubing near to the attached 20 ml syringe which is then removed and replaced with a tuberculin (1 ml) syringe containing gamete culture medium.

When a satisfactory aspirate volume is noted or no more aspirate is obtained, the needle is removed from the epididymis. The artery forceps that was used to clamp the end of the tubing is released. The aspirate is then flushed into a 1.5 ml sterile Eppendorf tube with culture medium from the attached tuberculin syringe. About 5 μl of the fluid in the Eppendorf tube is removed and placed on a clean dry glass slide before being examined under the microscope to ascertain the presence of live motile spermatozoa. The PESA procedure is repeated with fresh materials on that same epididymis and/or the opposite one until a satisfactory quantity of viable

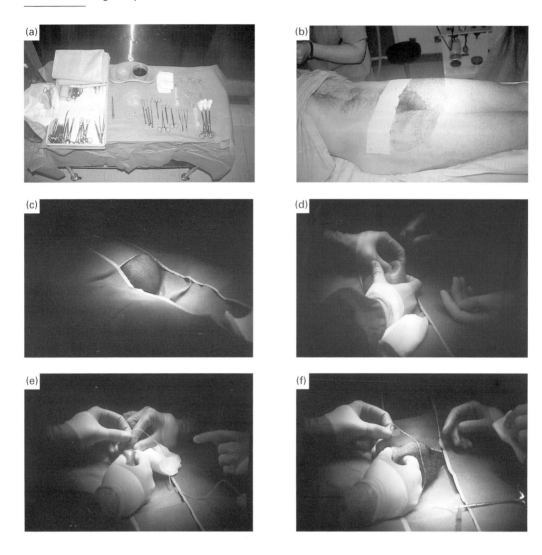

spermatozoa is deemed to have been recovered. It is not uncommon to recover sufficient spermatozoa for ICSI and freezing with the first puncture and aspiration, the procedure lasting less than 10 minutes. The samples are maintained at 37 °C while being transferred to the laboratory in a portable incubator. The patient is discharged home later that same day with a supply of simple analgesics. The sequence of events during PESA is shown in Figure 10.5.

PESA compared with MESA

PESA is a much simpler procedure compared with MESA and all the surgeon needs to learn is how to palpate and stabilize the epididymis for the needle

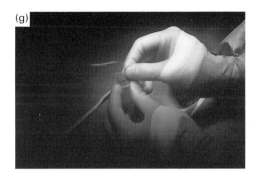
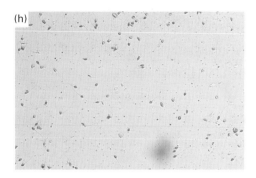

Figure 10.5 Highlights of the percutaneous epididymal sperm aspiration (PESA) procedure: (a) very few instrument requirements for PESA; (b) the skin is painted with antiseptics and the penis strapped away from the operation site; (c) sterile drapes are used to isolate the operating area; (d) the epididymis is palpated and stabilized with the fingers; (e) the needle is inserted into the epididymal mass and suction pressure applied with a 20 ml syringe; (f) the 20 ml syringe is replaced with a 1 ml syringe containing culture medium; (g) aspirated epididymal fluid is expelled into an Eppendorf tube; and (h) photomicrograph of a PESA sample showing spermatozoa, red blood cells, other types of cells and cellular debris.

insertion. PESA can be carried out under local anaesthesia in the majority of patients (Gorgy et al., 1997b). Since no scrotal incision is required postoperative pain is much less severe and almost non-existent in some cases. Most men are able to return to work the next day (Gorgy et al., 1997a). The PESA technique is much less prone to complications and continued evaluation of results has not revealed any significant complication (Meniru et al., 1998). PESA does not require the use of sophisticated equipment; only butterfly needles and a few non-toxic syringes are needed. As such PESA can be performed by any fertility specialist irrespective of whether he or she is a gynaecologist or urologist. The fact that the gynaecologist can carry out this procedure means that the goal of providing more holistic care for infertile couples will be better achieved with PESA than with MESA; both the man and his partner can be managed by the same clinician and there will be no need to move them from one department to another. Furthermore, PESA can be performed in a wide variety of settings and is potentially available to all assisted conception units at all times (Meniru et al., 1997a). The cost of PESA is much less than that of MESA.

The retrieval rate of spermatozoa with PESA is usually above 80% (Meniru et al., 1998) and the number of previous attempts does not appear to adversely affect the chances of future retrieval operations. This is most likely to be due to the fact that the scrotal incision of MESA causes adhesions and fibrosis around the epididymis

Table 10.3. Percutaneous epididymal sperm aspiration (PESA) compared with microepididymal sperm aspiration (MESA)

Variable	MESA	PESA
Scrotal incision required	Yes	No
Anaesthesia	General/local	Local/general
Technique	More complex	Simplified
Microsurgical equipment	Required	Not required
Surgeon	Uroandrologist	Any clinician
Objectives of holistic care	Not achieved	Better achieved
Potential for complications	More	Less
Postoperative pain	More	Less
Period of convalescence	Longer	Short
Cost of procedure	High	Much less
Availability to assisted conception units	Fewer units	Every unit
Overall sperm retrieval rate	Less/same	Higher/same
Outcome of ICSI with ejaculated spermatozoa	Similar	Similar

making it difficult for visual access to the epididymal tubules. Accruing evidence from PESA has not revealed any such scarring or scarring that is severe enough to impede access to the epididymal tubules (Meniru et al., 1998). It is doubtful if patients will agree to repeat MESA procedures if initial cycles of ICSI treatment do not result in pregnancy unlike the case with PESA. These differences are outlined in Table 10.3.

Vas deferens sperm aspiration

Spermatozoa can be aspirated from the vas deferens at the time of reversal of vasectomy. During vasectomy reversal, the blocked ends of adjacent segments of the vas deferens are reopened surgically. Fluid is aspirated from the segment that leads to the epididymis and testis. If examination of this fluid reveals spermatozoa this suggests that there is no blockage between that end of the vas deferens and the seminiferous tubules of the testis. Some surgeons aspirate as much of the fluid as possible and freeze the spermatozoa in case the vasectomy reversal operation is unsuccessful.

There have also been some reports of vas deferens sperm aspiration in patients with impotence. The operation involves a 4 cm scrotal incision to gain access to the vas deferens. The potential complications of this method of approach should be similar to that of MESA.

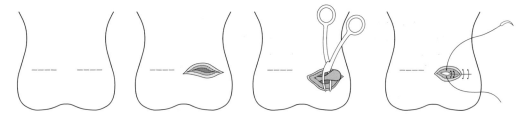

Figure 10.6 Testicular biopsy is the first stage of the testicular sperm extraction procedure.

Testicular sperm extraction (TESE)

This is another surgical sperm retrieval method and is applicable to a wide range of patients especially those in whom other retrieval techniques have been unsuccessful. TESE consists of testicular biopsy (Figure 10.6) and processing of the tissue samples to extract spermatozoa which are then used for ICSI. Pieces of testicular tissue are obtained during surgery and placed in dishes containing culture medium maintained at 37 °C. Back in the laboratory a range of techniques are available for use in liberating spermatozoa from the seminiferous tubules found in the testicular tissue specimen (Verheyan et al., 1995; Nagy et al., 1997; Meniru et al., 1998). Mechanical methods include gentle grinding of the tissue, squashing between glass slides, fine chopping with small sterile scissors, grating the tissue against a sieve or slitting individual seminiferous tubules with sharp needles under magnification. Chemical methods include the use of enzymes to digest the connective tissue matrix of the biopsy sample and haemolyzing buffers to eliminate the red blood cells that invariably contaminate the surgical specimen. This is a rapidly changing area of assisted reproduction technology. For example, patients with secretory azoospermia were previously thought to be irrevocably sterile. However, recent experience shows that careful examination of testicular tissue samples from these patients will reveal spermatozoa in a gratifyingly sizeable proportion of patients (Ben-Yosef et al., 1999). Even where mature spermatozoa cannot be found, spermatids are seen in up to 50% of cases and can be used for intracytoplasmic injection of the retrieved oocytes. Although the pregnancy rate with spermatid injection is presently low, continued improvement in technology will lead to more acceptable pregnancy rates (Edwards et al., 1994; Fishel et al., 1996; Mendoza & Tesarik, 1996; Tesarik & Mendoza, 1996; Tesarik et al., 1996).

Testicular biopsy has a complication profile that is similar to that of MESA namely bleeding, haematoma formation, infection, fibrosis and adhesion formation. A recent report has documented changes in testicular architecture and depression of testicular function following TESE especially when multiple biopsies are

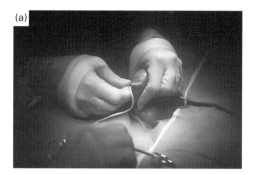

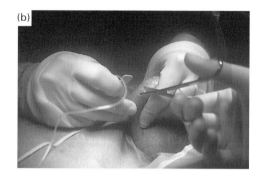

Figure 10.7 Testicular sperm aspiration: (a) a butterfly needle pierces the scrotal skin and used in sampling parts of the testis; and (b) a pair of clean sterile scissors is often required to cut a thread of testicular tissue stretching between the tip of the needle and scrotal skin, when withdrawing the needle from the testis at the end of the procedure.

taken (Schlegel & Su, 1997). This is a serious finding which should act to curb the over enthusiastic application of TESE (Meniru, 1998). Many patients who are subjected to TESE can be managed successfully by epididymal sperm aspiration. It is only those in whom this is not possible that TESE should be carried out. Finally, strong analgesics are required post-operatively and the patient needs to take time off work to recover. Many of these considerations led to the development of a less invasive alternative to TESE which is still compatible with successful outcome as described in the next section.

Testicular sperm aspiration (TESA)

TESA and PESA were both developed by the same team in the UK (Shrivastav et al., 1994; Craft & Shrivastav, 1994; Craft et al., 1995; Craft & Tsirigotis, 1995; Meniru et al., 1998). In TESA, a 19G butterfly needle is used in obtaining small strips of tissue from the testis (Figure 10.7). Suction is applied with an attached 20 ml syringe and in-and-out movements made with the needle without removing the tip from the substance of the testis. The retrieved tissue is flushed into sterile tubes with culture medium and taken to the laboratory for processing (Figures 10.8 & 10.9). The main method used in the laboratory is to slit individual seminiferous tubules using sizes 23–29G needles under magnification with the dissecting microscope. This liberates the contents of the tubules into the medium and further processing steps extract the spermatozoa from the sample. TESA has been applied successfully to cases of obstructive azoospermia and those with secretory azoospermia. The amount of testicular tissue available for processing is usually much smaller in the case of TESA unlike TESE but personnel usually adapt easily to the

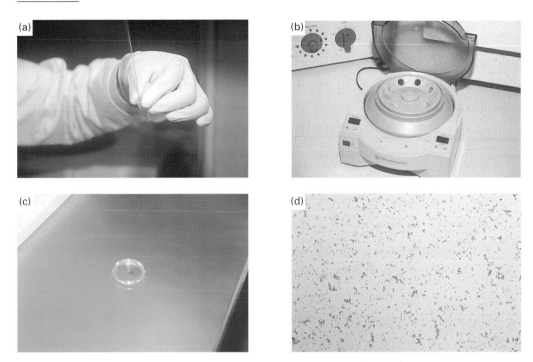

Figure 10.8 Laboratory aspects of testicular sperm aspiration (TESA): (a) the tissue specimen is washed with fresh culture medium; (b) a microcentrifuge allows the use of Eppendorf tubes and small volumes of culture medium; (c) after processing, the tissue sample is incubated until required for intracytoplasmic sperm injection later in the day; and (d) photomicrograph of processed TESA sample showing spermatozoa, red blood cells, other types of cells and cellular debris.

use of these small tissue samples. The number of spermatozoa extracted from TESA samples is usually more than required for immediate use and for freezing. Similar to PESA, TESA can be performed by a wide range of clinicians in a variety of settings and the patient is usually able to go back to work the following day.

In vitro culture of testicular tissue

As will be remembered from the first chapter, spermatozoa that are found in the testis and epididymis are not fully mature. Manifestations of physiological immaturity include immotility or exhibition of feeble shaking non-progressive movements. Testicular and epididymal spermatozoa have been used to establish several successful pregnancies. However, long-term follow-up study of the resulting progeny is required to ensure that the relative immaturity of the utilized spermatozoa does not impair their health, quality of life and life expectancy. Until that

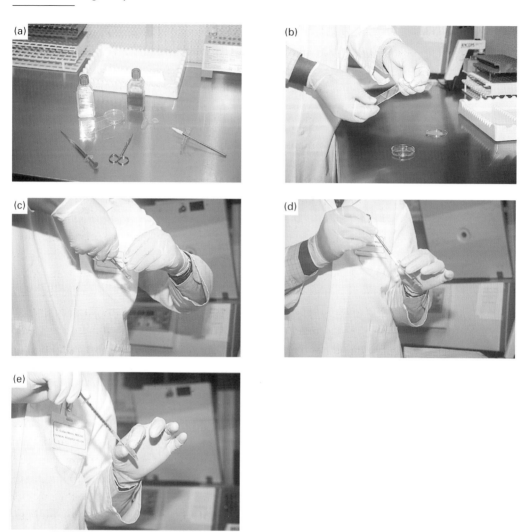

Figure 10.9 Techniques for liberating spermatozoa from the seminiferous tubules: (a) an overview of required equipment and materials; (b) testicular tissue being macerated between two clean sterile glass slides; (c) a pair of clean sterile scissors is used in chopping up the tissue sample; (d) the tissue can be ground with a pestle and mortar; and (e) testicular tissue and culture medium are drawn into a syringe through a 19G needle and expelled back into the Eppendorf tube through a size 23G needle. Another method is to identify individual seminiferous tubule segments with a dissecting microscope and slit them open with the sharp tip of a needle (not shown).

happens it is prudent to use mature spermatozoa for ICSI whenever possible. It is also important to ensure that only live spermatozoa are injected. Motility is one of the simplest ways of demonstrating viability of spermatozoa. While epididymal spermatozoa invariably show some form of motility this may not be readily evident in testicular spermatozoa. Furthermore, testicular spermatozoa tend to remain embedded or trapped within the surgical specimen and all these become important considerations in TESA because of the small volume of testicular tissue available for processing. A method for maturing human testicular spermatozoa in vitro has been developed and results in the acquisition of normal motility patterns by a sizeable proportion of spermatozoa following 24–72 hours of culture (Zhu et al., 1996).

Testicular tissue is obtained by the TESA technique as described previously. After withdrawing the needle from the testis, the aspirated testicular tissue is flushed into sterile centrifuge tubes with small volumes of culture medium and minced with a pair of clean sterile cutting scissors. Each seminiferous tubal segment is then slit with a needle. The tissue is washed twice with 5 ml of culture medium, centrifuging each time at $500 \times g$ for 10 minutes. The tissue pellet is placed in fresh droplets of culture medium and overlaid with equilibrated mineral oil. This is then incubated for 24–72 hours at 37 °C in a 5% CO_2-in-humidified-air mixture. The culture droplets are examined daily for evidence of sperm motility using an inverted phase contrast microscope (Figures 10.10 & 10.11).

It is likely that culture of testicular spermatozoa increases their maturity since there is a definite improvement in their motility pattern. The role of in vitro culture of testicular spermatozoa in assisted conception treatment programmes is still being defined. At present it is not applied to all cases where testicular spermatozoa are used for ICSI. In vitro culture is mainly used for those cases where the motility of freshly recovered testicular spermatozoa is non-existent. There have also been reports of in vitro culture of thawed frozen testicular tissue in order to stimulate motility of the spermatozoa.

Strategy for surgical sperm retrieval

Couples in whom azoospermia is diagnosed are evaluated to discover the exact cause of the problem. Investigations will include hormone assays aimed at finding out if there is evidence of testicular failure such as a raised concentration of follicle stimulating hormone. Vasography is performed in relevant cases. Both partners are offered screening for cystic fibrosis gene mutations in cases of CBAVD. In fact it is now advocated that all men with significant depression of their sperm parameters should have genetic counselling and chromosomal studies since accruing evidence suggests that some of them may have genetic disorders. Surgical sperm retrieval is

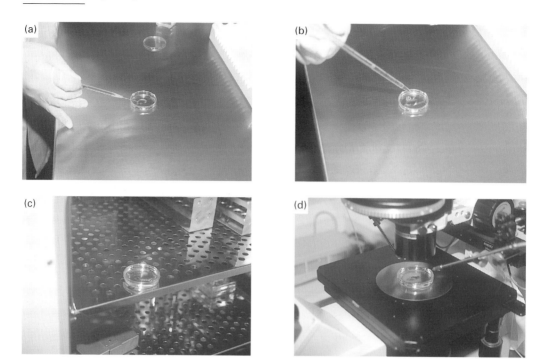

Figure 10.10 In vitro culture of testicular spermatozoa: (a) the processed tissue sample is placed in a droplet of culture medium; (b) the droplet is overlaid with 4 ml of washed and equilibrated liquid paraffin; (c) the dish is incubated for 24–72 hours at 37 °C in a 5% CO_2-in-humidified-air mixture; and (d) the culture droplet is examined daily for evidence of sperm motility using an inverted phase contrast microscope.

performed before making a final decision to carry out assisted conception treatment for couples. This preliminary retrieval operation acts as a diagnostic test, confirming the feasibility of surgical sperm retrieval for each patient. The particular retrieval method to be used depends on a number of considerations but the usual sequence should be PESA or MESA, TESA and/or TESE. TESA is carried out on failed PESA or MESA cases and TESE is best left as a back up procedure in case both PESA (or MESA) and TESA fail. The role of MESA in contemporary practice is unclear and is likely to remain solely within the realm of urologists.

Spermatozoa that are retrieved during the diagnostic procedure should be frozen in several plastic ampoules for use in subsequent treatment cycles thereby avoiding the need for repeat sperm retrieval (Tournaye et al., 1999). Testicular tissue can also be frozen prior to the extraction of spermatozoa provided a test sample yields spermatozoa on processing (Ben-Yosef et al., 1999). The frozen sample is thawed and processed on the day of oocyte aspiration or up to three days before that time. It is usual practice to carry out a test thaw of frozen spermatozoa or testicular tissue to

Figure 10.11 A motile testicular spermatozoon can be seen at the periphery of the culture droplet following incubation.

find out if they survive the procedure in acceptable numbers before committing a couple to assisted conception treatment.

Fresh PESA, MESA, TESA or TESE samples can be obtained on the day of egg collection if none was frozen beforehand. In these instances there is always a risk that no viable spermatozoa will be recovered. It is advisable to counsel patients, especially those who do not wish to have a preliminary diagnostic retrieval procedure, to consider the provision of donor spermatozoa as back up in case sperm retrieval fails on the crucial treatment day. This strategy is laid out in Figure 10.12.

Conclusion

Surgical sperm retrieval generally is a safe procedure and extends the range of treatment options available to infertile couples. Up-to-date evidence has not shown any procedure related abnormality in the children and the malformation rate is within the rate found in the general population. However, since some cases of male factor infertility may be related to genetic causes it follows that genetic disorders may be transferred to the progeny. All these should be explained in simple terms to the infertile couple who are then allowed enough time to decide on what they wish to

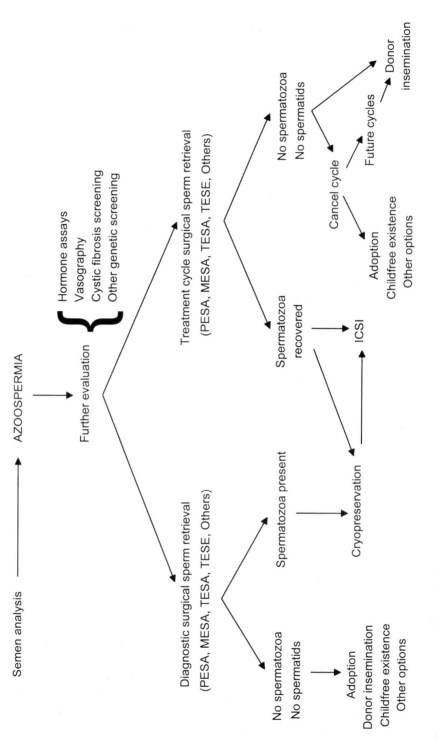

Figure 10.12 A strategy for surgical sperm retrieval in clinical practice.

be done. It is not within the remit of any member of the team to discourage genetically afflicted patients from seeking treatment using surgical sperm retrieval.

BIBLIOGRAPHY

Aboulghar, M. A., Mansour, R. T., Serour, G. I. et al. (1996). Prospective controlled randomized study of in vitro fertilization versus intracytoplasmic sperm injection in the treatment of tubal factor infertility with normal semen characteristics. *Fertility Sterility* **66**, 753–6.

Ben-Yosef, D., Yogev, L., Hauser, R. et al. (1999). Testicular sperm retrieval and cryopreservation prior to initiating ovarian stimulation as the first line approach in patients with non-obstructive azoospermia. *Human Reproduction* **14**, 1794–801.

Chillon, M., Casals, T., Mercier, B. et al. (1995). Mutations in the cystic fibrosis gene in patients with congenital absence of the vas deferens. *New England Journal of Medicine* **332**, 1475–80.

Craft, I. L. & Shrivastav, P. (1994). Treatment of male infertility. (Letter.) *Lancet* **344**, 191–2.

Craft, I. & Tsirigotis, M. (1995). Simplified recovery, preparation and cryopreservation of testicular spermatozoa. *Human Reproduction* **10**, 1623–7.

Craft, I., Tsirigotis, M., Bennett, V. et al. (1995). Percutaneous epididymal sperm aspiration and intracytoplasmic sperm injection in the management of infertility due to obstructive azoospermia. *Fertility and Sterility* **63**, 1038–42.

Devroey, P., Liu, J., Nagy, Z. et al. (1995). Pregnancies after testicular sperm extraction and intracytoplasmic sperm injection in non-obstructive azoospermia. *Human Reproduction* **10**, 1457–60.

Edwards, R. G., Tarin, J. J., Dean, N. et al. (1994). Are spermatid injections into human oocytes now mandatory? (Opinion.) *Human Reproduction* **9**, 2217–19.

Fishel, S., Aslam, I. & Tesarik, J. (1996). Spermatid conception: a stage too early, or a time too soon? (Opinion.) *Human Reproduction* **11**, 1371–5.

Gorgy, A., Meniru, G. I., Naumann, N. et al. (1997a). An evaluation of the efficacy of local anaesthesia for percutaneous epididymal sperm aspiration (PESA) and testicular sperm aspiration (TESA). *Journal of Assisted Reproduction and Genetics* **14** (Suppl.), 103S.

Gorgy, A., Naumann, N., Meniru, G. I. et al. (1997b). Postoperative morbidity following percutaneous epididymal sperm aspiration and/or testicular sperm aspiration under local anaesthesia. *Human Reproduction* **12** (Abstract book 1; P-016), 128.

Madgar, I., Seidman, S., Levran, D. et al. (1996). Micromanipulation improves in-vitro fertilization results after epididymal and testicular sperm aspiration in patients with congenital absence of the vas deferens. *Human Reproduction* **10**, 2151–4.

Mendoza, C. and Tesarik, J. (1996). The occurence and identification of round spermatids in the ejaculate of men with non-obstructive azoospermia. *Fertility and Sterility* **66**, 826–9.

Meniru, G. I. (1998). Time to rethink the indiscriminate application of testicular biopsy for sperm retrieval? *Human Reproduction* **13**, 505–6.

Meniru, G. I., Forman, R. G. & Craft, I. L. (1997a). Utility of percutaneous epididymal sperm aspiration in situations of unexpected obstructive azoospermia. *Human Reproduction* **12**, 1013–14.

Meniru, G. I., Gorgy, A., Podsiadly, B. T. & Craft, I. L. (1997b). Results of percutaneous epididymal sperm aspiration and intracytoplasmic sperm injection in two major groups of patients with obstructive azoospermia. *Human Reproduction* **12**, 2443–6.

Meniru, G. I., Gorgy, A., Batha, S. et al. (1998). Studies of percutaneous epididymal sperm aspiration (PESA) and intracytoplasmic sperm injection. *Human Reproduction Update* **4**, 57–71.

Meniru, G. I., Tsirigotis, M., Zhu, J. J. & Craft, I. (1996). Successful percutaneous epididymal sperm aspiration (PESA) after more than 20 years of acquired obstructive azoospermia. *Journal of Assisted Reproduction and Genetics* **13**, 449–50.

Mercier, B., Verlingue, C., Lissens, W. et al. (1995). Is congenital bilateral absence of vas deferens a primary form of cystic fibrosis? Analyses of the CFTR gene in 67 patients. *American Journal of Human Genetics* **56**, 272–7.

Nagy, Z. P., Verheyen, G., Tournaye, H. et al. (1997). An improved treatment procedure for testicular biopsy specimens offers more efficient sperm recovery: case series. *Fertility Sterility* **68**, 376–9.

Schlegel, P. N., Cohen, J., Goldstein, M. et al. (1995). Cystic fibrosis gene mutations do not affect sperm function during in vitro fertilization with micromanipulation for men with bilateral congenital absence of vas deferens. *Fertility and Sterility* **64**, 421–6.

Schlegel, P. N. & Su, L.-M. (1997). Physiological consequences of testicular sperm extraction. *Human Reproduction* **12**, 1688–92.

Shrivastav, P., Nadkarni, P., Wensvoort, S. & Craft, I. (1994). Percutaneous epididymal sperm aspiration for obstructive azoospermia. *Human Reproduction* **9**, 2058–61.

Shtainer, A. & Nagler, H. M. (1995). Surgical treatment of male infertility. In *Infertility Evaluation and Treatment*, ed. W. R. Keye, Jr., R. J. Chang, R. W. Rebar & M. R. Soules, pp. 621–51. Philadelphia: W. B. Saunders Company.

Silber, S. J., Van Steirteghem, A. C., Liu, J. et al. (1995). High fertilization and pregnancy rate after intracytoplasmic sperm injection with spermatozoa obtained from testicle biopsy. *Human Reproduction* **10**, 148–52.

Temple-Smith, P. D., Southwick, G. J., Yates, C. A. et al. (1985). Human pregnancy by in-vitro fertilization (IVF) using sperm aspirated from the epididymis. *Journal of In Vitro Fertilization and Embryo Transfer* **2**, 119–22.

Tesarik, J. & Mendoza, C. (1996). Spermatid injection into human oocytes. I. Laboratory techniques and special features of zygote development. *Human Reproduction* **11**, 772–9.

Tesarik, J., Rolet, F., Brami, C. et al. (1996). Spermatid injection into human oocytes. II. Clinical application in the treatment of infertility due to non-obstructive azoospermia. *Human Reproduction* **11**, 780–3.

Tournaye, H., Merdad, T., Silber, S. et al. (1999). No differences in outcome after intracytoplasmic sperm injection with fresh or with frozen-thawed epididymal spermatozoa. *Human Reproduction* **14**, 90–5.

Tournaye, H., Verheyen, G., Nagy, P. et al. (1997). Are there any predictive factors for successful testicular sperm recovery in azoospermic patients? *Human Reproduction* **12**, 80–6.

Van Steirteghem, A. C., Nagy, P., Joris, H. et al. (1996). The development of intracytoplasmic sperm injection. *Human Reproduction* 11 (Suppl. 1), 59–72.

Verheyan, G., De Croo, I., Tournaye, H. et al. (1995). Comparison of four mechanical methods to retrieve spermatozoa from testicular tissue. *Human Reproduction* 10, 2956–9.

Zhu, J. J., Tsirigotis, M., Pelekanos, M. & Craft, I. L. (1996). In-vitro maturation of human testicular spermatozoa. (Letter.) *Human Reproduction* 11, 231–2.

11

Intratubal replacement of gametes and embryos (GIFT, ZIFT)

Introduction

Contrary to popular belief, the development of infertility treatment options has not been such a radical exercise. There have always been attempts to pattern treatment modalities as closely as possible to the natural situation and reduce interference to a minimum. This is in part due to uncertainty of what the optimal in vitro situation should be and the impact of the intervention on the viability and integrity of the gametes, embryos, pregnancy or resulting progeny. A classic example is male factor infertility, in which several more conservative and less effective treatment options were utilized for several years before the advent of intracytoplasmic sperm injection (ICSI) (see Chapter 9). Conventional in vitro fertilization (IVF) treatment was developed to overcome the sterilizing effect of tubal blockage. Although the merits of the treatment were obvious, it was still felt that some women with non-tubal infertility may benefit from a less radical approach; the retrieved oocytes were mixed with a prepared sperm sample and replaced in the fallopian tubes, thereby allowing fertilization and subsequent events to take place within the natural environment of the body. Another driving force for the development of tubal gamete or embryo replacement techniques was the then lack of confidence of the in vitro culture environment, including the culture medium and the various aspects of laboratory processing of gametes and embryos. Gamete intrafallopian transfer (GIFT) was popularized by Ricardo H. Asch from the USA while tubal replacement of fertilized eggs, called zygote intrafallopian transfer (ZIFT), was pioneered by Paul Devroey and his colleagues in Belgium. ZIFT now covers all other acronyms that have been used in the past to describe similar or related procedures such as ProST, TET, TEST and SET (see Appendix).

Gamete intrafallopian transfer (GIFT)

Indications

The group of patients proposed initially as suitable candidates for GIFT were those with unexplained infertility. The spectrum of patients later widened to include

Table 11.1. Patient groups who have been treated with gamete intrafallopian transfer

Unexplained infertility
Endometriosis
Male factor problems
Immunological infertility (antisperm antibodies)
Failed donor insemination
Older women
Pelvic adhesions with patent fallopian tubes

those with all other causes of infertility, except bilateral tubal blockage (Table 11.1). There is always a chance that a couple with unexplained infertility may have subtle defects in the functioning of their reproductive system but assisted conception treatment has generally been found to produce good results in this group of patients. Apparently, superovulation and bringing the gametes in close contact within the lumen of the fallopian tube is enough to overcome many of the putative defects in couples during treatment with GIFT.

There is still much that is unknown about endometriosis, but the fact that GIFT has been found to be successful in a significant proportion of patients who have at least one patent tube confirms the nebulous relationship between the disorder and infertility. GIFT is one of the treatment options that has been evaluated for use in couples with some degree of male factor associated infertility. Variable results were documented by various workers but the availability of ICSI and adoption of a more pragmatic approach to the management of male factor infertility patients has virtually eliminated this indication for GIFT. GIFT has been performed in patients who have minor pelvic adhesions but patent tubes. This group of patients, however, have a high incidence of ectopic pregnancy (14.3–33%) if GIFT is successful compared to those with no pelvic adhesions (4–5%) (references in Brinsden & Asch, 1992). Intratubal pathology may exist in these females and GIFT should be applied with caution. Immunological infertility arising from the presence of antisperm antibodies in the female genital tract may not be optimally treated by performing GIFT because the same interference with normal fertilization may still be found following intratubal transfer of sperm and retrieved oocytes. In the same vein conventional IVF or ICSI may be more appropriate for patients with seminal antisperm antibodies, because of the need to document the fertilization potential of sperm from these patients.

Usually, artificial insemination is the method of choice for women who require the use of donor sperm and do not have any obvious female factor problem that precludes its application. However, some may not become pregnant after many cycles of donor insemination. The question then arises as to what is responsible for the repeated failure and whether conventional IVF or GIFT should be carried out as the next option. Some workers have reported excellent results following GIFT in such women; pregnancy rates of 50% and above have been reported.

Women aged 40 years and above are known to have significantly reduced fertility potential, primarily due to oocyte ageing, and this becomes even more obvious during assisted conception treatment. Results have generally been found to be poor in this group of patients but in a review by Weckstein & Asch (1993) these women seem to have an improved outcome following GIFT. However, as the authors rightly point out, treatment with donor oocytes may be a better option for some of these women, especially in the face of rising pre-treatment follicle stimulating hormone levels and other evidence of impending menopause. A possible reason for an improved outcome following GIFT in comparison to conventional IVF treatment in older women, if indeed it is true, is that the physiological tubal environment prevents hardening of the zona pellucida. This allows normal hatching of the blastocyst from the zona pellucida prior to implantation unlike the situation when there is increased hardening of the zona pellucida which is thought to be more common when in vitro culture is carried out. Very good results have been achieved in older women who have GIFT with donor oocytes from younger women. However, this is not an exclusive preserve of GIFT because similar heightened pregnancy rates are found following IVF treatment in older women using oocytes donated by younger women.

Ovarian stimulation

Superovulation is carried out using principles and techniques that have been described in Chapter 8. In summary, pituitary down regulation and desensitization are brought about using any of the commercially available gonadotrophin releasing hormone agonists (GnRHa). Ovarian stimulation is carried out by administering two ampoules or more of gonadotrophin preparations daily for about 14 days (range 12–21). Ovarian response to stimulation is monitored mainly with ultrasound scanning although some clinicians may include serial assays of serum oestradiol and other hormones. When a satisfactory number of developing follicles reach a diameter of 18–22 mm an ovulation triggering injection of 10 000 IU of human chorionic gonadotrophin is administered and oocyte retrieval scheduled for 34–36 hours later (Meniru & Craft, 1997; Meniru et al., 1997). The man is required to produce a sample of semen about two hours before oocyte retrieval to allow adequate time for sperm preparation in the laboratory. Obviously, the man must have had a full semen analysis before this time.

Oocyte retrieval

In earlier years oocyte retrieval for GIFT and indeed for conventional IVF treatment was mainly by laparoscopy (Figure 11.1) and occasionally laparotomy or

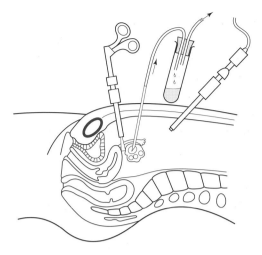

Figure 11.1 Laparoscopic oocyte retrieval.

minilaparotomy. Transvaginal ultrasound guided oocyte retrieval is now the most popular technique and results in the retrieval of a larger proportion of the retrievable oocytes found within developing ovarian follicles when compared to other routes of oocyte retrieval. Furthermore, ultrasound guidance allows emptying of most ovarian follicles through fewer punctures on the ovarian surface. This reduces the morbidity of the procedure and the amount of blood loss into the abdominal cavity from the puncture wounds on the ovarian surface. The morphology and maturity of each retrieved oocyte are graded during the procedure and the three best oocytes selected for transfer. As was noted in Chapter 8, the number of oocytes or embryos to be replaced depends on medical opinion, patients' choice and legislation in the particular country.

Intrafallopian transfer of oocytes and sperm

The selected oocytes are picked up with the transfer catheter together with a volume of the prepared sperm suspension that contains about 100 000 sperm. Care is taken to avoid the transfer of a large volume of fluid; the total volume of transferred gametes and fluid should not exceed 30–50 µl. Laparoscopy has been the main route utilized for the replacement of oocytes and sperm during the GIFT procedure (Table 11.2) (Figure 11.2). The abdominal cavity is distended with a volume of 100% carbon dioxide gas to allow the safe introduction of the laparoscope and other instruments, and easy visualization of the abdominal and pelvic organs. Following this, some workers will replace the gas with a mixture containing 5% carbon dioxide, 5% oxygen and 90% nitrogen because of fears that the 100% carbon dioxide may be toxic to the gametes. However, it has not been proven

Table 11.2. Approaches for gamete intrafallopian transfer

Laparoscopy
Minilaparotomy
Transcervical (transvaginal)
Culdoscopy

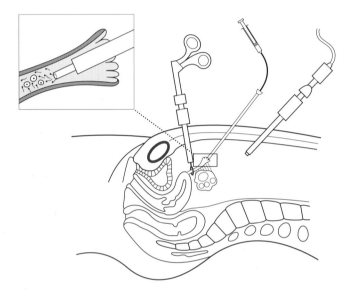

Figure 11.2 GIFT (gamete intrafallopian transfer) being performed under laparoscopic guidance.

conclusively that this has a significant effect on the pregnancy rate and many clinicians still use 100% carbon dioxide with equally good results. Following insertion of the laparoscope into the abdominal cavity the pelvic organs are inspected and if blood stained fluid is found anywhere in the pelvis it is aspirated. The best looking and most accessible fallopian tube is gently cannulated with a guide catheter (cannula).

It is important to reduce exposure of the gametes to room temperature to a minimum otherwise certain structures in the oocyte called the spindle apparatus may become disrupted. The spindle apparatus is important for an orderly separation of chromosomes whenever a cell divides. A team approach produces best results; there should be synchronization of activities and an experienced embryologist can load the gametes in the transfer catheter within a few seconds. This means that the guide catheter has to be introduced into the fallopian tube before the gametes are brought out of the incubator and loaded into the transfer catheter. The transfer catheter is gently introduced into the guide catheter to enter the fallopian

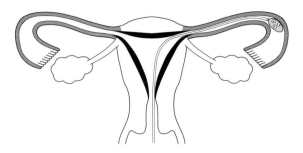

Figure 11.3 Transcervical tubal cannulation and GIFT (gamete intrafallopian transfer) being performed.

tube for a distance of about 4 cm. The gametes are gently ejected into the fallopian tube using positive pressure generated with the attached syringe. The guide catheter is first removed gently from the fallopian tube before gently removing the transfer catheter. The transfer catheter is then handed over to the embryologist to check for retention of oocytes in the catheter. Afterwards, some but not all clinicians may place part of the remaining sperm sample from the patient's partner in the cervical canal (intracervical insemination), the logic being that this provides a continuous supply of sperm to the fallopian tubes (Weckstein & Asch, 1993).

In previous years there was uncertainty as to whether all selected oocytes should be transferred into one fallopian tube or split into two groups and transferred into both tubes. Current evidence does not support such a protocol and it is possible that the increased operative time may exert its own deleterious effects on gamete quality. Moreover tubal catheterization may cause intratubal trauma, infection or inflammation (Tournaye et al., 1996), so it is best to restrict any potential damage to one tube if possible.

Other routes that have been used during GIFT are shown in Table 11.2. Minilaparotomy involves making a small incision (1–3 cm) in the lower part of the anterior abdominal wall between the umbilicus and the upper part of the mons pubis. This allows limited access to the ovaries, fallopian tubes and surrounding organs. Culdoscopy involves making a small incision in the posterior fornix of the vagina and the introduction of a culdoscope to visualize the fallopian tubes, ovaries and pelvic organs. Cannulation of the fallopian tubes and some surgical operations can be carried out during culdoscopy. Minilaparotomy and culdoscopy have never achieved world-wide popularity and are rarely performed nowadays for GIFT.

It is also possible for a transcervical cannulation of the fallopian tubes and GIFT to be performed (Figure 11.3). Tubal cannulation is achieved by hysteroscopic guidance, transvaginal ultrasound control or falloscopy. Alternatively, a blind 'tactile' technique can be used. Although some enthusiasts have reported good results with transcervical tubal cannulation and GIFT, the general experience is that these latter techniques do not have associated pregnancy rates that are similar to those achieved with the laparoscopic approach. The reasons for this are not clear but may include the use of wrong techniques, trauma to the endometrium, and the mucous membrane of the fallopian tubes during cannulation.

Conventional IVF of excess oocytes

If there are more oocytes than required for immediate transfer they are inseminated with calculated volumes of the prepared sperm suspension after some hours of incubation in the laboratory. The inseminated oocytes are assessed after about 18 hours for signs of fertilization. Normally fertilized eggs are frozen on that same day, at the pronuclear stage, or the following day, when cleavage must have started.

Aftercare

Luteal phase support can also be carried out using daily intramuscular progesterone injections, intravaginal progesterone gel (Crinone), progesterone pessaries (Cyclogest) or hCG injections as described in Chapter 8. As noted in Chapter 8, the dose of Cyclogest varies amongst different practitioners but a common dose regimen is 400 mg inserted twice a day for 12–14 days, at the end of which a serum β-hCG pregnancy test is performed. If a positive pregnancy test result is obtained progesterone supplementation is continued until a total of 8–12 weeks of pregnancy. An ultrasound scan is performed three weeks following the positive pregnancy test and repeated at the gestational age of 12 weeks when the patient is then referred for antenatal care.

Zygote intrafallopian transfer (ZIFT)

One of the criticisms of the GIFT technique is that the events of fertilization and early embryo development are hidden from view in the fallopian tubes. As such it is not possible to ascertain how well these events occur when no pregnancy results. This consideration becomes more important for couples where there is a risk of failed fertilization or poor fertilization rates such as in those with male factor problems or female antisperm antibodies. Attempts have been made to predict the fertilization rate of transferred oocytes by documenting the outcome of conventional IVF carried out on the excess oocytes. Although conflicting results were reported by various workers the predominant feeling is that IVF results with supernumerary oocytes do not correlate well with the subsequent outcome of the GIFT treatment.

The various post-fertilization tubal replacement techniques were developed in response to these concerns. Conventional IVF is used to generate fertilized (two pronucleate) eggs which are then transferred; the question of fertilization potential thereby being resolved. If there is uncertainty of the cleavage pattern and quality of the resulting embryos, transfer can be delayed for another 24 hours so as to allow the first two embryo cleavage divisions to occur. Although various acronyms have been used in the past, ZIFT is now accepted as a suitable blanket terminology for all tubal transfers of pronucleate eggs or embryos.

Indications for ZIFT have varied but include immunological infertility, male factor infertility, previous failure to become pregnant following GIFT, use of donor oocytes and retrieval of predominantly immature oocytes. The results of studies that compared the pregnancy rates associated with ZIFT and IVF-ET (IVF-intrauterine embryo transfers) treatments are summarized by Tournaye et al. (1996). A secondary analysis of those results showed a median pregnancy rate, per gamete or embryo replacement cycle, of 38% (range 14–58%) for ZIFT and 27% (range 12–55%) for IVF-ET.

Treatment outcome following GIFT and ZIFT compared to IVF

Comparative analysis of treatment results following GIFT, ZIFT and conventional IVF-ET is a confusing exercise. On the one hand, national registries and many centres have reported pregnancy and delivery rates for intratubal transfers that are at least one and a half times or even twice that of IVF-ET or more. On the other hand, an almost equal number of centres achieve results which do not show much of an advantage of intratubal transfers over IVF-ET. Several reports in which this issue has been discussed end up invoking nebulous confounding factors that may be responsible for the inconsistency of results and state that the two study populations (GIFT/ZIFT and IVF-ET) may not be comparable in many respects. Furthermore, centres that initially reported results much in favour of GIFT and ZIFT, in later years have seen the margin largely disappear as results from IVF-ET have caught up. One obvious factor is the general improvement of in vitro culture conditions resulting from a greater understanding of gamete/embryo nutritional requirements, improved gamete and embryo handling techniques, and the availability of more efficient incubators.

Kenny (1995) reported on the results of a detailed search of the published literature on outcome of GIFT, TEST, ProST and IVF-ET treatment. She compared the results derived from 216 papers published between 1987 and 1992 with figures from some national registers (Table 11.3). GIFT consistently outperformed IVF-ET in all outcome categories that were analysed and similar trends were noted in all sources of treatment outcome data. A category is shown in Table 11.3 for illustration purposes. TEST and ProST were not compared because of small numbers. This review is quite authoritative and is probably the best and least biased source of such comparative data on outcome of these treatments.

Table 11.3. Comparative analysis of pregnancy rates following gamete intrafallopian transfer (GIFT) and in vitro fertilization-intrauterine embryo transfer (IVF-ET)

	Clinical pregnancy rates per oocyte/embryo transfer	
	IVF-ET (%)	GIFT (%)
Amalgamated literature rates	23.88 (SD 11.64)	32.38 (SD 19.70)
National registers		
Australia (1988)	16.8	27.7
USA (1989)	21	30
Australia (1989)	16.5	29.3
Australia (1990)	16.7	29.2

Notes:
The number of reports in the amalgamated literature was 156 for the IVF-ET group and 64 for the GIFT group.
Source: Adapted from Kenny (1995).

The role of GIFT/ZIFT in present day infertility treatment

What then is the role of intratubal replacement of gametes or embryos in contemporary assisted conception practice? The answer depends on the experience of each assisted conception unit and their results. If a large proportion of treatment being carried out in a particular unit consists of GIFT and/or ZIFT, and they obtain very good results – results that justify the additional expense, invasiveness and post-operative morbidity associated with these procedures (except possibly transcervical tubal cannulation and gamete or embryo transfer) – then the unit should continue offering the treatment to well-selected patients after discussion of alternatives.

If, however, fewer GIFT/ZIFT procedures are performed in a unit and associated pregnancy rates are similar to or even less than those obtained from IVF-ET in the same unit, then GIFT/ZIFT is probably best reserved for certain groups of patients such as: (1) those with proven cervical stenosis or in whom cervical cannulation is very difficult or impossible in the index or previous IVF treatment cycle; (2) women who return after previous successful GIFT or ZIFT treatment and wish to have the same treatment; (3) patients having frozen embryo transfer, with the hope that the natural environment of the fallopian tubes will ameliorate the deleterious effect of cryopreservation on embryo quality; (4) in women aged 40 years and above who insist on having assisted conception treatment with their own oocytes; and (5) those whose religious doctrine suggest GIFT or ZIFT as more acceptable alternatives to IVF-ET.

Another possible indication for GIFT is diagnostic or therapeutic laparoscopy in women who have been shown, using hysterosalpingography, to have patent fallopian tubes. Superovulation in such cases is ideally carried out with clomiphene citrate so that ovarian enlargement is not great thereby making it easy for the visualization of the pelvis and manipulation of the pelvic organs during the laparoscopy. Reports have shown that it is possible to examine the pelvis adequately and perform adhesiolysis and destruction of endometriotic tissue and still have a pregnancy rate of between 24–35%. Cycle cancellation may be more frequent here, from premature luteinizing hormone surge, since pituitary suppression with GnRHa is not carried out in these patients. Alternatively, ovulation induction can be carried out after pituitary suppression using smaller doses of gonadotrophin injections to stimulate the growth of fewer follicles.

Conclusion

Intratubal placement of gametes and embryos is one of the major advances of modern infertility treatment and has resulted in the birth of several thousand children. The development of these techniques was partly stimulated by shortcomings of the then in vitro culture system. Some of those early problems with in vitro culture have now been resolved and better systems are being developed to allow intrauterine transfer of blastocysts after extended in vitro culture. It is therefore pertinent that questions may be asked regarding the utility of the continued practice of GIFT and ZIFT. Often the best response to such questions is that of waiting for future developments in assisted reproduction technology, since they will provide better answers.

BIBLIOGRAPHY

Asch, R. H., Ellsworth, L. R, Balmaceda, J. P. & Wong, P. C. (1984). Pregnancy after translaparoscopic gamete intra fallopian transfer. *Lancet* 2, 1034–5.

Balmaceda, J. P., Manzur, A. & Asch, R. H. (1995). Gamete intrafallopian transfer. In *Infertility Evaluation and Treatment*, ed. W. R. Keye, R. J. Chang, R. W. Rebar & M. R. Soules, pp. 772–9. Philadelphia: W. B. Saunders Company.

Brinsden, P. R. & Asch, R. H. (1992). Gamete intrafallopian transfer. In *A Textbook of In Vitro Fertilization and Assisted Reproduction*, ed. P. R. Brinsden & R. H. Asch, pp. 227–36. Carnforth: Parthenon Publishing.

Bulletti, C. (1996). Debating tubal transfer in assisted reproductive technologies. *Human Reproduction* 11, 1820–2.

Craft, I. & Al-Shawaf, T. (1992). IVF versus GIFT. *Journal of In Vitro Fertilization and Embryo Transfer* 9, 424–7.

Craft, I. & Brinsden, P. (1989). Alternatives to IVF: the outcome of 1071 first GIFT procedures. *Human Reproduction* 4, 29–36.

Devroey, P., Braekmans, P., Smitz, J. et al. (1986). Pregnancy after translaparoscopic zygote intrafallopian transfer in a patient with sperm antibodies. *Lancet* 1, 1329.

Jansen, R. P. & Anderson, J. C. (1987). Catheterisation of the fallopian tubes from the vagina. *Lancet* 2, 309.

Kenny, D. T. (1995). In vitro fertilization and gamete intrafallopian transfer: an integrative analysis of research, 1987–1992. *British Journal of Obstetrics and Gynaecology* 102, 317–25.

Menezo, Y. J. R. & Janny, L. (1996). Is there a rationale for tubal transfer in human ART? *Human Reproduction* 11, 1818–20.

Meniru, G. I. & Craft, I. L. (1997). Ovarian stimulation for the assisted reproduction technologies. In *A Handbook of Intrauterine Insemination*, ed. G. I. Meniru, P. R. Brinsden & I. L. Craft, pp 56–76. Cambridge: Cambridge University Press.

Meniru, G. I., Tsirigotis, M. & Craft, I. L. (1997). Controlled superovulation for intrauterine insemination. In *A Handbook of Intrauterine Insemination*, ed. G. I. Meniru, P. R. Brinsden & I. L. Craft, pp 77–96. Cambridge: Cambridge University Press.

Tournaye, H., Camus, M., Ubaldi, P. et al. (1996). Is there still a role for tubal transfer procedures? *Human Reproduction* 11, 1815–18.

Weckstein, L. N. & Asch, R. H. (1993). Gamete intrafallopian transfer, zygote intrafallopian transfer, tubal embryo transfer, and beyond. In *Assisted Reproductive Technologies*, ed. R. P. Marrs, pp. 68–88. Boston: Blackwell Scientific Publications.

12

Intrauterine insemination

Introduction

Intrauterine insemination (IUI) is an assisted conception treatment method that can be used for the alleviation of infertility in certain groups of patients. It involves the deposition of a washed sample of sperm in the uterine cavity around the predicted time of ovulation. Usually the woman's ovaries are also simultaneously stimulated to produce two to four oocytes. These manipulations have certain advantages over the natural situation. Firstly, many more sperm are spared from destruction in the vagina and they are directly placed in the uterine cavity. Secondly, the distance which sperm have to travel to reach the site of fertilization in the fallopian tube is greatly shortened. Thirdly, more oocytes are available in the fallopian tubes and this increases the chances of at least one of them being fertilized. Finally, the presence of more than one embryo likewise improves the chances of one of them implanting successfully in the uterus. IUI is one of the simpler and less expensive assisted conception treatment methods. Its effectiveness is such that it is now regarded as a suitable first line assisted conception treatment for most infertile couples with patent fallopian tubes (van Voorhis 1997). The conduct of IUI will be discussed in the following sections. Details on how to set up and run an effective IUI service can be found in a comprehensive tome on the subject (Meniru et al., 1997).

Trends in artificial insemination

Artificial insemination with partner or donor sperm has been practiced for more than 200 years. For most of that time the insemination technique was intravaginal (Table 12.1, Figure 12.1); freshly produced semen was deposited as high up in the vagina as possible using a syringe or similar device. The problem with this method of insemination is that of uncertainty about the number of spermatozoa that enter the cervical canal and ultimately reach the site of fertilization in the fallopian tubes. It is estimated that only about 1% of sperm succeed in doing so following normal

Table 12.1. Artificial insemination techniques

Intravaginal insemination
Peri-cervical insemination
Intracervical insemination
Intrauterine insemination
Direct intraperitoneal insemination
Direct intrafollicular insemination
Intratubal insemination

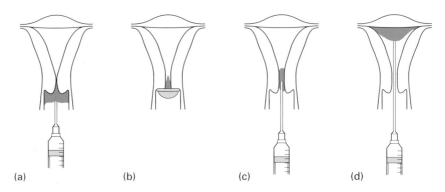

Figure 12.1 The 'minimally invasive' artificial insemination techniques: (a) intravaginal insemination; (b) pericervical insemination; (c) intracervical insemination; and (d) intrauterine insemination.

sexual intercourse and ejaculation into the vagina. Furthermore, the destructive effects of vaginal acidity may become overwhelming for small volume semen samples. These considerations probably led to the development of other insemination techniques such as peri-cervical, intracervical and intrauterine insemination (Figure 12.1b–d). Peri-cervical insemination involves placing the semen sample in a cap-like device which is then fitted over the cervix as shown in Figure 12.1 (b). This allows closer contact between the semen sample and the cervical os. The cap-like device also shields the sperm contained in the semen sample from the acidic vaginal environment. For intracervical insemination less than 0.5 ml of the semen sample is carefully injected into the cervical canal. Again there is still uncertainty about the number of sperm that succeed in reaching the uterus and fallopian tubes from these points of deposition.

Early attempts at IUI using the raw unprocessed ejaculate were not encouraging as patients invariably had severe and painful uterine cramps following the procedure. This was due to strong uterine contractions stimulated by prostaglandins that

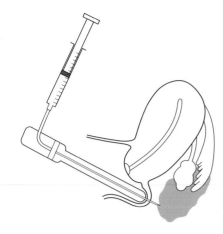

Figure 12.2 Performance of direct intraperitoneal insemination under guidance using ultrasound scanning.

are contained in semen. The incidence of infection was also higher. These considerations led to a reduction of interest in the intrauterine route of insemination. There was however a resurgence of interest in IUI following the development of in vitro fertilization (IVF) because the latter procedure involves the use of a 'washed' semen sample that is usually devoid of most of the chemical constituents of semen such as prostaglandins, and other cellular debris including dead sperm and white blood cells. Deposition of washed sperm samples in the uterine cavity rarely causes uterine cramps except if a large volume of fluid is injected rapidly and under high pressure.

More invasive artificial insemination techniques have since been developed but they have not enjoyed as much popularity as the less invasive methods. Examples of invasive insemination techniques include direct intraperitoneal insemination (DIPI) (Figure 12.2), direct intrafollicular insemination and intratubal insemination. DIPI involves the injection of a washed sperm sample through the posterior fornix of the vagina and into the peritoneal cavity. It can be done under guidance of ultrasound scanning. However, a multicentre study did not demonstrate a significant difference between the pregnancy rates following DIPI as compared with IUI (Ajossa et al., 1997). Direct intrafollicular insemination is carried out by injecting a washed sperm sample into an ovarian follicle that is programmed to rupture and ovulate at the time of injection or shortly afterwards. This procedure can also be carried out through the vagina under ultrasound scanner guidance similar to the procedure of oocyte aspiration for IVF treatment. Intratubal insemination can be carried out by passing a cannula through the cervical canal, uterine cavity and into the fallopian tube where a washed sperm sample is deposited. Cannulation of the

Table 12.2. Contraindications to intrauterine insemination

Blocked tubes and other tubal pathology
Genital tract infection in either partner
Severely abnormal semen parameters
Genetic abnormality in husband
Unexplained genital tract bleeding
Pelvic mass
Older woman
Co-existing multiple infertility aetiologies
Pelvic surgery
Pregnancy contraindicated
Severe illness in one or both partners
Recent chemotherapy or radiotherapy
Multiple failures at intrauterine insemination

Source: Adapted from Meniru et al. (1997).

fallopian tube can be carried out blindly relying on tactile sensation and the use of pre-shaped cannulas that adapt to the contours of the upper genital tract as they ascend and eventually 'find' the opening of the fallopian tube into the uterine cavity. Alternatively tubal cannulation can be performed under visual guidance with a hysteroscope that is introduced into the uterine cavity through the cervical canal.

Patient selection

Contraindications

Couples should be evaluated as described in earlier chapters before deciding on whom should have IUI treatment. One of the reasons for this is to identify those who have contraindications to the proposed treatment (Table 12.2). Women with blockage of both tubes obviously cannot become pregnant with IUI treatment because of the requirement of normal functioning fallopian tubes. Although some clinicians carry out IUI in women with only one patent tube it is not clear how effective treatment is in such women. This is because whatever caused the blockage or the loss of the other tube might have also caused some damage to the remaining, apparently patent, tube. This may interfere with normal mechanisms following IUI such that either no pregnancy occurs or if it occurs, movement of the embryo(s) down the fallopian tube may become arrested possibly resulting in ectopic pregnancy. The same reasoning applies to women who have patent fallopian tubes in the presence of post-infection pelvic adhesions. Women with ovarian failure should have IVF treatment with donor oocytes. Couples in which the men have severe sperm abnormalities should not have IUI treatment because of uncertainty regarding the ability of the sperm to fertilize the oocyte. What constitutes severe sperm abnormality is relative but some studies have shown that the results of IUI are less favourable when the total number of inseminated actively moving sperm is less than one million (Ombelet et al., 1995; Campana et al., 1996). What is probably required here is experience and compassion for the couple. If the practitioner believes that IVF or intracytoplasmic sperm injection (ICSI) treatment is more appropriate for a particular couple they should be advised accordingly. The fact that there are anecdotal reports of pregnancies in couples with unfavourable prognostic features should not be a reason for recommending IUI treatment to similar couples. Couples with complex infertility problems need a more pragmatic treatment approach such as IVF since it is possible to better document the manner of response of the patient to each stage of the treatment until after embryo transfer. This is unlike in IUI where events such as the number and quality of ovulated oocytes, fertilized eggs and the resulting embryos cannot be documented. It is only by selecting out poor prognosis patients as defined above that the true efficacy of IUI becomes apparent. Finally, it must be stressed that the age of the woman is one of the factors that weigh heavily on the mode of management chosen for infertile couples. More effective treatment options such as IVF are chosen over others, such as IUI, when the woman's age is of concern. In other words, when the period available to a couple for achieving optimal results following treatment is restricted by the woman's age, IVF will be the most suitable treatment to use. However, there is no magic line demarcating 'young' and 'older' women and there is no guarantee of the exact length of remaining optimal reproductive functioning for each particular woman. Based on population statistics, the rate of decline of female fertility begins to accelerate after the age of 35 years and the fertility of the woman plummets after 40 years of age. It follows that infertility treatment should be more pragmatic in women who present to the clinicians at age 35 years and above. Other contraindications listed in Table 12.2 are self explanatory.

Indications

Having eliminated contraindications to the use of IUI for fertility treatment it becomes easier to identify patients who may benefit from the treatment. Male and female factor problems have been respectively described in Chapters 4 and 5 and are listed in Tables 12.3–12.5. These should be reviewed in relation to the following sections.

Insemination with fresh partner sperm

Some men with impotence or ejaculatory problems can be managed successfully using techniques and medications that are described in Chapter 7. Emission of

Table 12.3. Male factor problems that are amenable to treatment with intrauterine insemination

Using fresh partner sperm
Retrograde ejaculation
Impotence or ejaculatory dysfunction
Hypospadias
Hypospermia
Non-liquefying or highly viscous sperm
Subnormal sperm parameters
Seminal antisperm antibodies
Unexplained infertility

Using frozen partner sperm
Absentee husband
Anti-cancer treatment in the man
Vasectomy
Poor sperm parameters
Other drug therapy

Table 12.4. Female factor problems that are amenable to treatment with intrauterine insemination

Vaginismus
Cervical factor problem
Ovulatory dysfunction
Allergy to seminal plasma
Endometriosis
Unexplained infertility

Source: Adapted from Meniru et al. (1997).

Table 12.5. Indications for intrauterine insemination using donor sperm

Azoospermia of primary testicular origin
Severely subnormal semen parameters
Hereditary disease in the man
Rhesus isoimmunization
Repeated failure at IVF or ICSI treatment
Single woman
Lesbian

Notes:
IVF: in vitro fertilization; ICSI: intracytoplasmic sperm injection.
Source: Adapted from Meniru et al. (1997).

semen can be stimulated in those with intractable problems by the use of rectal electrostimulation or penile vibration and the sample prepared for IUI. In retrograde ejaculation the urine is alkalinized by giving the patient sodium bicarbonate orally some hours before ejaculation. The patient then urinates into a container or a catheter used to empty the bladder. The sample is prepared immediately to remove the sperm from the potentially toxic environment in urine. Patients with other intractable ejaculatory problems can collect the semen sample in containers following masturbation.

IUI treatment can also be used for couples in whom the man has a mild depression of seminal parameters (Cohlen et al., 1998). Treatment can be successful for this group of patients but if the degree of depression becomes significant, IVF is required to document retention of optimal fertilization rates. If this is assured by this 'diagnostic' IVF cycle and the patient does not become pregnant during that cycle subsequent treatment could be by IUI, IVF or gamete intrafallopian transfer (GIFT).

Men with seminal antisperm antibodies may have reduced fertility but infertility is not invariable. An attempt at IUI may be made in well-informed consenting patients, but IVF or even ICSI may be more appropriate for those with severe varieties of the problem. IUI has been a traditional indication for women with cervical hostility (see Chapter 5) as it bypasses the cervix and deposits the sperm within the uterine cavity. However, some women with antisperm antibodies in their cervical secretions could also be producing these antibodies in secretions found higher up in the genital tract including the fallopian tubes but these females may not be easily identifiable.

Intractable vaginismus is another traditional indication for artificial insemination. The woman could even inseminate herself by performing intravaginal insemination using a sterile syringe. Her partner ejaculates into a sterile container and the sample drawn up with the syringe. IUI can also be carried out for these patients, especially if several attempts at intravaginal insemination without ovarian stimulation do not result in pregnancy. There may still be problems with inserting the speculum and other instruments required for IUI due to the patient being unable to relax her vaginal wall muscles. A combination of sedation and the use of nitrous oxide gas (laughing gas) may be adequate for these patients but there must be consent from the couple and the clinician must be documented to have been chaperoned during the insemination procedure. It is conceivable that a few patients may require general anaesthesia for this to be carried out although the author is not aware of anywhere this has happened.

A large proportion of women with treatable ovulatory problems can be managed successfully by using drugs such as clomiphene citrate or gonadotrophin injections. Others may be treated by dietary manipulations and weight gain or loss. Many of those who then ovulate can become pregnant following timed sexual intercourse. For those who do not become pregnant after a reasonable length of time, say 6–12 months, IUI can be offered as the next treatment option.

The relationship between endometriosis and infertility is not clear especially in cases of mild to minimal disease. The decision to offer treatment to the couple may not relate to the extent of the disease but more to other factors that have been discussed in other chapters such as the age of the woman, length of infertility and whether they wish to have treatment. IUI may be carried out in the presence of mild disease but the advisability of carrying out the treatment in women with moderate and especially severe disease is a moot point; IVF may be a better option for the latter group of women especially after some months of suppressive treatment using gonadotrophin releasing hormone agonists (GnRHa).

Unexplained infertility may not be completely 'unexplained' as some of these patients will be shown later to have subtle defects in their reproductive functions. However, it appears that IUI, just like other assisted conception treatment methods such as IVF and GIFT, overcomes some of the defects and results in pregnancy. This is probably due to stimulation of the ovaries, production of more than one oocyte, increase in the density of spermatozoa in the vicinity of the oocyte(s) and the availability of more than one embryo for implantation. Studies have shown a good outcome of treatment using IUI in this group of patients (Hannoun et al., 1998; Trout & Kemmann, 1999).

Allergy to semen has been reported as a rare indication for IUI with washed sperm (Shapiro et al., 1981). The patient became pregnant after seven cycles of natural cycle IUI treatment and delivered twin babies.

Insemination with frozen partner sperm

Although fresh or frozen partner sperm samples can be utilized for IUI when treating patients with infertility problems that were described above, there are particular indications for the specific use of frozen partner semen (Table 12.3). Infrequent sexual intercourse may occur when partners live apart for a significant length of their time together, such as shift workers, those in business and people who have to travel out of their place of domicile for work. However, these living arrangements may not necessarily lead to infertility unless there is already an existing fertility problem even if it is subtle. If such couples seek fertility treatments such as IUI, the man may be required to have his semen frozen and stored at the treatment unit prior to the start of treatment. The same can be done for a couple of whom the partner is in prison.

Semen is increasingly being frozen for men who have testicular and other cancers and require removal of the testes, chemotherapy and/or radiotherapy of the testes.

These are essentially sterilizing treatment options although testicular function can recover when certain classes of cytotoxic drugs are used. Other patients may have to be treated long-term with drugs that are known to depress sperm production such as sulphasalazine and niridazole (Forman et al., 1996). Prior storage of the patients' semen will allow the man a chance at biological parenthood if he survives the disease and treatment. IUI is an option that can be tried provided the semen parameters of the frozen thawed sample are satisfactory. If not, IVF or ICSI can be carried out.

Men who are contemplating having vasectomy for permanent contraception may elect to have their semen stored in case they ever decide to have more children in the future. This is not an unreasonable behaviour because studies have shown that a significant proportion of men and woman who are sterilized regret it afterwards. Others may divorce and remarry or some of their children may die and they then wish to have more. IUI provides a relatively low cost, minimally invasive avenue for achieving parenthood in such conditions.

An uncommon indication is the pooling of semen samples produced by the same man over a period of time to compensate for subnormal sperm parameters (Aboulghar et al., 1991). The required number of ampoules of frozen sperm are then thawed and prepared for use in IUI treatment. With the recent availability of more effective treatment options for men with significantly depressed sperm parameters, such as ICSI, this indication is not likely to be used much in the coming years except if the couple insist on having IUI, or new scientific evidence shows that it has associated pregnancy rates similar to those of ICSI treatment.

Insemination with donor sperm

Donor sperm samples are required to be frozen, in countries with relevant edicts, for at least six months to enable retesting of the donor for disease status especially in relation to the human immunodeficiency virus infection. In previous years, donor insemination was the only realistic treatment option that was available for patients with azoospermia and other situations of severe depression of semen parameters that were not amenable to drug or surgical treatment (Table 12.5). Nowadays surgical sperm retrieval and ICSI can be applied successfully to patients who can afford the treatment. There still remains a core group of patients in whom sperm retrieval is unsuccessful and require the use of donor sperm for their partners to become pregnant. There are other patients who may opt for donor insemination rather than the use of the still novel treatment techniques or when repeated attempts at IVF or ICSI fail. Others may not be able to afford the more expensive treatment with ICSI. Donor sperm could be used for procreation in couples where the man has a serious hereditary disease whose transmission to

Table 12.6. Ovarian cycle management for intrauterine insemination

Natural ovarian cycle
CC
CC + gonadotrophins
Gonadotrophins
GnRHa + gonadotrophins

Notes:
CC: clomiphene citrate; GnRHa: gonadotrophin releasing hormone agonist

progeny is undesirable. However, the advent of pre-implantation genetic diagnosis (Chapter 15) has now made it possible for even some of these couples to become genetic parents. Similarly, severe Rhesus isoimmunization may have been an indication in the past for donor insemination but nowadays gestational surrogacy (Meniru & Craft, 1997) will allow the affected woman to have children; IVF is carried out using her oocytes and the husband's sperm and the resulting embryos transferred to a gestational carrier. Finally, single women and lesbian couples are increasingly asking for donor insemination.

Ovarian cycle management

Artificial insemination can be carried out during the natural ovarian cycle or following ovarian stimulation. Various ovarian cycle management regimens that have either been used in the past or are still being used are shown in Table 12.6. Clomiphene citrate (CC) tablets are administered at a dose of 50–100 mg once daily from Days 2–6 of the menstrual cycle, i.e. for five days. This regimen may initially lead to the development of some follicles in the ovary but only one usually continues to grow and ovulation of one oocyte usually occurs. The addition of gonadotrophin injections in the latter half of the follicular phase may encourage more of the follicles to continue to develop with the eventual ovulation of more than one oocyte. It is felt that the availability of more than one oocyte for fertilization improves the chance of conception. Some women may not respond to CC or are not suitable candidates for ovulation induction using CC. Such women are administered gonadotrophin injections from Day 2 of the menstrual cycle or on the second day of a withdrawal bleed following pre-treatment with progesterone preparations or combined oral contraceptive tablets. The dose of gonadotrophin injection is usually 75–150 IU administered daily or every other day. The last regimen involves the use of GnRHa, as described in Chapter 8, to prevent a premature surge of luteinizing hormone (LH) secretion by the pituitary gland.

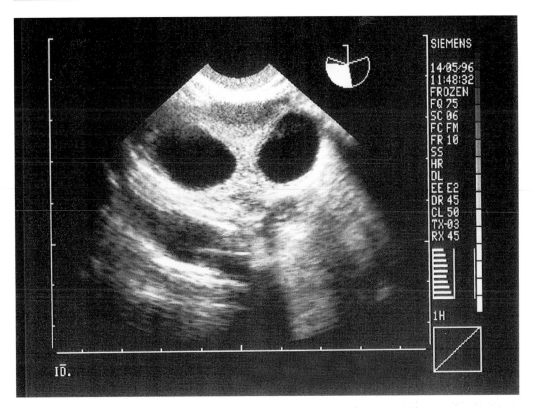

Figure 12.3 Transvaginal sonogram: ovary showing multiple follicular development in response to superovulation induction. This is preparatory to intrauterine insemination and the aim is for production of three and certainly not more than five mature fertilizable oocytes. Adapted from Meniru et al. (1997).

Monitoring of follicular development and predicting ovulation

Ultrasound scanning provides the most practical method for monitoring follicular development during IUI treatment (Figure 12.3). The follicle becomes visible using transvaginal ultrasound scanning by the time its diameter is between 2 and 3 mm. Its growth is usually linear and the diameter increases by 2–3 mm per day. Ovulation occurs when the follicular diameter reaches 18–24 mm. Ultrasound scanning will also demonstrate progressive thickening of the endometrial layer, which ideally should be more than 9 mm thick (Figure 12.4). Monitoring ovarian response to stimulation by serial oestradiol assays is not very useful during IUI treatment as the ultrasound provides adequate evidence of follicular growth.

The other component of monitoring during IUI treatment is prediction of the time of ovulation. This is most important in treatment cycles where GnRHa is not used to suppress pituitary activity leading to the possibility of an LH surge. This

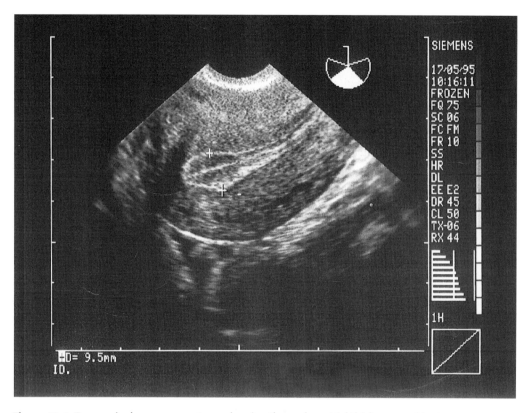

Figure 12.4 Transvaginal sonogram: uterus showing the endometrial thickness and texture.

surge may occur before the follicle has reached the required diameter of 18–24 mm. In fact, the surge can occur any time after the follicular diameter exceeds 16 mm. If this surge is not detected the woman may ovulate before her next monitoring session. Urinary LH home detection kits are commonly used once the follicular diameter exceeds 15–16 mm. Another way of determining when to start monitoring for LH is by estimating the average day of ovulation, by reviewing the woman's previous menstrual cycles' length, and commencing urine testing four days before that time. If the LH surge is detected the woman is immediately administered an injection of 10 000 IU of human chorionic gonadotrophin (hCG) injection to support that surge. The LH surge that occurs during ovarian stimulation may not be as high as would normally occur during the natural cycle. Moreover, the amount of LH produced may not be adequate to induce the necessary final maturational changes in all oocytes if more than one follicle develops in the ovary. The LH surge may occur in up to 20% of cycles during IUI treatment. For the remaining patients an injection of 10 000 IU of hCG is administered once the diameter of the leading follicle reaches 18 mm or more. As has been stated in an earlier chapter hCG shares key structural similarities with LH and can induce similar maturational changes in the oocyte.

The timing of insemination

IUI is timed to occur as close to ovulation as possible. Since the actual moment of ovulation is rarely known or witnessed, knowledge of the time-course relationship between the LH surge or administration of hCG and ovulation is important. Ovulation normally occurs about 40–45 hours after the onset of the LH surge (Lenton, 1993). Not all follicles ovulate at the same time; rather they do so in waves. These considerations have led some clinicians to carry out insemination twice, separated by 24 hours, around the time of ovulation. The first insemination is carried out 24 hours after administering hCG injection and repeated 24 hours later. For patients who mount a spontaneous LH surge, hCG is administered and the first insemination carried out immediately following detection of the surge. The immediate insemination is due to the uncertainty of the exact interval between the onset of the LH surge and its detection. In such instances the second insemination may be optionally carried out 24 hours after the first one. There is no agreement amongst practitioners regarding the timing and optimal number of inseminations to be carried out during one treatment cycle (Centola et al., 1990; Lenton, 1993; Brook et al., 1994; Ransom et al., 1994; Khalifa et al., 1995). Some advocate one insemination while others perform the procedure twice and a few clinicians perform insemination three or more times during the cycle. The more accurate the monitoring methods used, the fewer the number of required inseminations since the time of ovulation will be known with greater certainty.

The insemination procedure

The semen sample is prepared as described for IVF treatment in Chapter 8. The volume of the prepared sperm sample should be restricted to 1 ml although some clinicians prefer a smaller volume and others use larger volumes of up to 4 ml. A comprehensive account of these techniques is presented in the book by Meniru et al. (1997) as they are beyond the scope of the present chapter. A simple technique for IUI is as follows, and the equipment requirement is usually minimal (Figure 12.5).

The woman lies in the lithotomy position (which approximates to lying on her back with the knees and hips flexed and thighs spread apart). A warm speculum is moistened with warm sterile water and gently inserted in the vagina to expose the cervix and cervical os. The cervix is gently wiped with several cotton wool balls soaked in normal saline solution. The insemination cannula is attached to the 1 ml syringe and used in drawing up the sperm suspension. The cannula is then gently introduced into the uterine cavity through the cervical canal and the sperm suspension gently expelled (Figure 12.1). All instruments are withdrawn and the patient

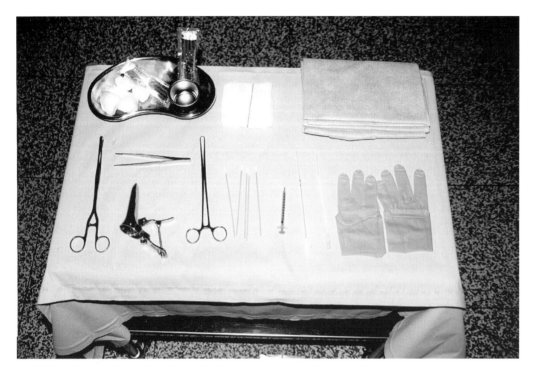

Figure 12.5 A simple instrument set-up for intrauterine insemination.

allowed to lie on the procedure couch for some minutes before going home. A pregnancy test is carried out about two weeks later.

Success rates

About 10–15% of couples will become pregnant in each cycle of treatment. Higher pregnancy rates of up to 34.3% have been reported by some workers (Ajossa et al., 1997). Most couples who get pregnant using IUI do so within the first four cycles of treatment. These four cycles can often be completed within a period of 8–12 months. It is not advisable to continue treatment with IUI after this number of attempts. Instead, the patient should have IVF treatment if she is still not pregnant.

Complications

Complications are not common following treatment with IUI. Pelvic infection may occur in 0.01–0.2% of couples. Allergic reaction to albumin, antibiotics or some other components of the sperm culture medium can occur but this is rare (Sonenthal et al., 1991; Smith et al., 1992). The incidence of multiple pregnancy is increased (11–30% of pregnancies) because the ovaries are stimulated to produce more than one oocyte and there is no control over the number of resulting embryos that implant. The ovaries may become overstimulated in about 1% of cases leading to ill health, which may last for two weeks or more. This is called ovarian hyperstimulation syndrome. It is not yet clear if IUI leads to the formation of antisperm antibodies in the female. Studies have documented an increase in the titre of blood borne antisperm antibodies in already sensitized women following IUI (Kremer, 1979). The incidence of miscarriage is between 20 and 30% and the ectopic pregnancy rate is 3–5.5%; these rates are similar to those obtained following IVF and other assisted conception treatments (Ombelet et al., 1995).

Some studies have suggested that the risk of developing ovarian cancer is higher in women who have ovarian stimulation (Whittemore, 1993). This issue is far from resolved since several reports have produced conflicting findings. What is known with a reasonable degree of certainty is that most women who have infertility treatment involving ovarian stimulation do not develop ovarian cancer later in life. There are a number of possibilities regarding the aetiology of cancer in these women and their prior use of ovarian stimulants. Ovarian stimulation may have (a) no effect at all; (b) a negative (protective) effect; (c) a direct positive (enhancing) effect; (d) an indirect positive effect mediated through elaboration of carcinogens; and (e) an uncertain effect which depends on interaction with modulators such as type and duration of infertility, genetic influences, environmental and lifestyle factors, oral contraceptive usage, pregnancies, breast-feeding and ovulatory age.

Conclusion

IUI now has an established role as a low risk, low cost, front line, assisted conception treatment method. Its efficacy is enhanced when patients are carefully screened to avoid treating those with contraindications such as suspected tubal disease. Cumulative data has shown that making four attempts at IUI before resorting to IVF treatment is a reasonable strategy (Martinez et al., 1993). Cost-effectiveness studies support this approach at managing infertile couples (van Voorhis et al., 1997).

BIBLIOGRAPHY

Aboulghar, M. A., Mansour, R. T., Serour, G. I. et al. (1991). Cryopreservation of the occasionally improved semen samples for intrauterine insemination: a new approach in the treatment of idiopathic male infertility. *Fertility and Sterility* **56**, 1151–5.

Ajossa, S., Melis, G. B., Ciani, A. et al. (1997). An open multicenter study to compare the efficacy of intraperitoneal insemination and intrauterine insemination following multiple follicular development as treatment for unexplained infertility. *Journal of Assisted Reproduction and Genetics* **14**, 15–20.

Berger, G. S. (1987). Intratubal insemination. *Fertility and Sterility* **48**, 328–30.

Brinsden, P. R., Wada, I., Tan, S. L. et al. (1995). Diagnosis, prevention and management of ovarian hyperstimulation syndrome. *British Journal of Obstetrics and Gynaecology* **102**, 767–72.

Brook, P. F., Barratt, C. L. R. & Cooke, I. D. (1994). The more accurate timing of insemination with regard to ovulation does not create a significant improvement in pregnancy rates in a donor insemination program. *Fertility and Sterility* **61**, 308–13.

Campana, A., Sakkas, D., Stalberg, A. et al. (1996). Intrauterine insemination: evaluation of the results according to the woman's age, sperm quality, total sperm count per insemination and life table analysis. *Human Reproduction* **11**, 732–6.

Centola, G. M., Mattox, J. H. & Rauberts, R. F. (1990). Pregnancy rates after double versus single insemination with frozen donor semen. *Fertility and Sterility* **54**, 1089–92.

Chung, C. C., Fleming, R., Jamieson, M. E. et al. (1995). Randomized comparison of ovulation induction with or without intrauterine insemination in the treatment of unexplained infertility. *Human Reproduction* **10**, 3139–41.

Cohlen, B. J., te Velde, E. R., van Kooij, R. J. et al. (1998). Controlled ovarian hyperstimulation and intrauterine insemination for treating male subfertility: a controlled study. *Human Reproduction* **13**, 1553–8.

Crosignani, P. G. & Walters, D. E. (1994). Clinical pregnancy and male subfertility, the ESHRE multicentre trial on the treatment of male subfertility. *Human Reproduction* **9**, 1112–18.

Crosignani, P. G., Walters, D. E. & Soliani, A. (1991). The ESHRE multicentre trial on the treatment of unexplained infertility: a preliminary report. *Human Reproduction* **6**, 953–8.

Fanchin, R., Olivennes, F., Righini, C. et al. (1995a). A new system for fallopian tube sperm perfusion leads to pregnancy rates twice as high as standard intrauterine insemination. *Fertility and Sterility* **64**, 505–10.

Fanchin, R., Olivennes, F., Righini, C. et al. (1995b). A new system for fallopian tube sperm perfusion leads to pregnancy rates three times as high as standard IUI in cases of sperm abnormalities. *15th World Congress on Fertility and Sterility,* Montpellier, France, 17–22 September 1995.

Fishel, S. & Jackson, P. (1989). Follicular stimulation for high tech pregnancies: are we playing it safe? *British Medical Journal* **299**, 309–11.

Forman, R., Gilmour-White, S. & Forman, N. (1996). *Drug Induced Infertility and Sexual Dysfunction.* Cambridge: Cambridge University Press.

Friedman, A. J., Juneau-Norcross, M. & Sedensky, B. (1991). Antisperm antibody production following intrauterine insemination. *Human Reproduction* **6**, 1125–8.

Friedman, A. J., Juneau-Norcross, M., Sedensky, B. et al. (1992). Life-table analysis of intrauterine insemination pregnancy rates for couples with cervical factor, male factor and idiopathic infertility. *Fertility and Sterility* **55**, 1005–7.

Glezerman, M. (1993). Artificial insemination. In *Infertility: Male and Female,* ed. V. Insler & B. Lunenfeld, 2nd edn, pp. 643–58. Edinburgh: Churchill Livingstone.

Golan, A., Herman, A., Soffer, Y. et al. (1994). Ultrasonic control without hormone determination for ovulation induction in in-vitro fertilization/embryo transfer with gonadotrophin-releasing hormone analogue and human menopausal gonadotrophin. *Human Reproduction* 9, 1631–3.

Hannoun, A., Abu-Musa, A., Kaspar, H. & Khalil, A. (1998). Intrauterine insemination: the effect of ovarian stimulation and infertility diagnosis on pregnancy outcome. *Clinical and Experimental Obstetrics and Gynecology* 25, 144–6.

Harris, R., Whittemore, A. S., Intyre, J. & the Collaborative Ovarian Cancer Group (1992). Characteristics relating to ovarian cancer risk: collaborative analysis of 12 US case-control studies. III. Epithelial tumors of low malignant potential in white women. *American Journal of Epidemiology* 136, 1204–11.

Horn-Ross, P. L., Whittemore, A. S., Intyre, J. & the Collaborative Ovarian Cancer Group (1992). Characteristics relating to ovarian cancer risk: collaborative analysis of 12 US case-control studies. VI. Non-epithelial cancers among adults. *Epidemiology* 3, 490–5.

Jansen, R. P. S., Anderson, J. C., Radonic, I. et al. (1988). Pregnancies after ultrasound-guided fallopian insemination with cryostored donor semen. *Fertility and Sterility* 49, 920–2.

Junior, J. G. F., Baruffi, R. L. R., Mauri, A. L. & Stone, S. C. (1992). Radiological evaluation of incremental intrauterine instillation of contrast material. *Fertility and Sterility* 58, 1065–7.

Karande, V. C., Rao, R., Pratt, D. E. et al. (1995). A randomized prospective comparison between intrauterine insemination and fallopian sperm perfusion for the treatment of infertility. *Fertility and Sterility* 64, 638–40.

Khalifa, Y., Redgement, C. J., Tsirigotis, M. et al. (1995). The value of single versus repeated insemination in intra-uterine donor insemination cycles. *Human Reproduction* 10, 153–4.

Kremer, J. (1979). A new technique for intrauterine insemination. *International Journal of Fertility* 24, 53–60.

Lenton, E. A. (1993). Ovulation timing. In *Donor Insemination*, ed. C. L. R. Barratt & I. D. Cooke, pp. 97–110. Cambridge: Cambridge University Press.

Li, T. C. (1993). A simple, non-invasive method of fallopian tube sperm perfusion. *Human Reproduction* 8, 1848–50.

Lucena, E., Ruiz, J. A., Mendoza, J. C. et al. (1989). Vaginal intratubal insemination (VITI) and vaginal GIFT, endosonographic technique: early experience. *Human Reproduction* 4, 658–62.

Makler, A., DeCherney, A. & Naftolin, F. (1984). A device for injecting and retaining a small volume of concentrated spermatozoa in the uterine cavity and cervical canal. *Fertility and Sterility* 42, 306–8.

Marshburn, P. B. & Kutteh, W. H. (1994). The role of antisperm antibodies in infertility. *Fertility and Sterility* 61, 799–811.

Martinez, A. R., Bernardus, R. E., Vermeiden, J. P. W. & Schoemaker, J. (1993). Basic questions on intrauterine insemination: an update. *Obstetrical and Gynecological Survey* 48, 811–28.

Meniru, G. I. & Craft, I. L. (1997). Experience with gestational surrogacy as a treatment for sterility resulting from hysterectomy. *Human Reproduction* 12, 51–4.

Meniru, G. I., Brinsden, P. R. & Craft, I. L. (Eds) (1997). *A Handbook of Intrauterine Insemination*. Cambridge: Cambridge University Press.

Recommended chapters in the text
- Brinsden, P. R. & Marcus, S. F. (Chapter 1). An overview of intrauterine insemination, pp. 1–8.
- Meniru, G. I. & Hutchon, S. P. (Chapter 2). Equipment, design and organisation of the unit, pp. 9–22.
- Meniru, G. I. & Akagbosu, F. T. (Chapter 3). Patient selection and management, pp. 23–45.
- Raeburn, A. R. & Meniru, M. O. (Chapter 4). Fertility counselling, pp. 46–55.
- Meniru, G. I. & Craft, I. L. (Chapter 5). Ovarian stimulation for the assisted reproduction technologies, pp. 56–76.
- Meniru, G. I., Tsirigotis, M. & Craft, I. L. (Chapter 6). Controlled superovulation for intrauterine insemination, pp. 77–96.
- Meniru, G. I. & Craft, I. L. (Chapter 7). Ultrasonography in the managment of infertility with special reference to intrauterine insemination, pp. 97–128.
- Fleming, S., Meniru, G. I., Hall, J. A. & Fishel, S. (Chapter 8). Semen analysis and sperm preparation, pp. 129–45.
- Meniru, G. I. & Brinsden, P. R. (Chapter 9). Intrauterine insemination techniques, pp. 146–58.
- Bynoe, F. E. (Chapter 10). The role of the nurse in an insemination programme, pp. 159–162.
- Green, S. & Fleming, S. D. (Chapter 11). Principles and practice of semen cryopreservation, pp. 163–89.
- Crich, J. P. (Chapter 12). Donor sperm banking, pp. 190–206.
- Meniru, G. I. (Chapter 13). Complications of superovulation and intrauterine insemination, pp. 207–23.
- Meniru, G. I. (Chapter 14). Concluding remarks: thoughts on the management of infertility, pp. 234–41.

Mortimer, D. (1994). *Practical Laboratory Andrology*. New York: Oxford Universtiy Press.

O'Herlihy, C., Pepperell, R. J. & Robinson, H. P. (1982). Ultrasound timing of human chorionic gonadotrophin administration in clomiphene stimulated cycles. *Obstetrics and Gynecology* **59**, 40–5.

Ombelet, W., Puttemans, P. & Bosmans, E. (1995). Intrauterine insemination: a first-step procedure in the algorithm of male subfertility treatment. *Human Reproduction* **10** (Suppl. 1), 90–102.

Plosker, S. M., Jacobson, W. & Amato, P. (1994). Predicting and optimizing success in an intrauterine insemination programme. *Human Reproduction* **9**, 2014–21.

Pratt, D. E., Bieber, E., Barnes, R. et al. (1991). Transvaginal intratubal insemination by tactile sensation: a preliminary report. *Fertility and Sterility* **56**, 984–6.

Ransom, M. X., Blotner, M. B., Bohrer, M. et al. (1994). Does increasing frequency of intrauterine insemination improve pregnancy rates significantly during superovulation cycles? *Fertility and Sterility* **61**, 303–7.

Remohi, J., Gastaldi, C., Patrizio, P. et al. (1989). Intrauterine insemination and controlled ovarian hyperstimulation in cycles before GIFT. *Human Reproduction* **4**, 918–20.

Ripps, B. A., Minhas, B. S., Carson, S. A. & Buster, J. E. (1994). Intrauterine insemination in fertile women delivers larger numbers of sperm to the peritoneal fluid than intracervical insemination. *Fertility and Sterility* **61**, 398–400.

Roger, A., Lalich, D. O., Edward, L. et al. (1988). Life table analyses of intrauterine insemination pregnancy rates. *American Journal of Obstetrics and Gynecology* **158**, 980–4.

Rossing, M. A., Daling, J. R., Weiss, N. S. et al. (1994). Ovarian tumors in a cohort of infertile women. *New England Journal of Medicine* **331**, 771–6.

Sacks, P. C. & Simon, J. A. (1991). Infectious complications of intrauterine insemination: a case report and literature review. *International Journal of Fertility* **36**, 331–9.

Schenker, J. G. & Ezra, Y. (1994). Complications of assisted reproductive techniques. *Fertility and Sterility* **61**, 411–22.

Shapiro, S. S., Kooistra, J. B., Schwartz, D. et al. (1981). Induction of pregnancy in a woman with seminal plasma allergy. *Fertility and Sterility* **36**, 405–7.

Smith, Y. R., Hurd, W. W., Menge, A. C. et al. (1992). Allergic reactions to penicillin during in vitro fertilization and intrauterine insemination. *Fertility and Sterility* **58**, 847–9.

Sonenthal, K. R., McKnight, T., Shaughnessy, M. A. et al. (1991). Anaphylaxis during intrauterine insemination secondary to bovine serum albumin. *Fertility and Sterility* **56**, 1188–91.

Trout, S. W. & Kemmann, E. (1999). Fallopian sperm perfusion versus intrauterine insemination: a randomized controlled trial and metaanalysis of the literature. *Fertility and Sterility* **71**, 881–5.

Tsirigotis, M., Hutchon, S., Yazdani, N. & Craft, I. (1995). The value of oestradiol estimations in controlled ovarian hyperstimulation cycles. (Letter.) *Human Reproduction* **10**, 972–3.

van Voorhis, B. J., Sparks, A. E. T., Allen, B. D. et al. (1997). Cost-effectiveness of infertility treatments: a cohort study. *Fertility and Sterility* **67**, 830–6.

Venn, A., Watson, L., Lumley, J. et al. (1995). Breast and ovarian cancer incidence after infertility and in vitro fertilization. *Lancet* **346**, 995–1000.

Whittemore, A. S. (1993). Fertility drugs and the risk of ovarian cancer. *Human Reproduction* **8**, 999–1000.

Whittemore, A. S., Harris, R., Intyre, J. & the Collaborative Ovarian Cancer Group (1992). Characteristics relating to ovarian cancer risk: collaborative analysis of twelve US case-control studies. II. Invasive epithelial ovarian cancer in white women. *American Journal of Epidemiology* **136**, 1184–203.

Willemsen, W., Kruitwagen, R., Bastiaans, B. et al. (1993). Ovarian stimulation and granulosa-cell tumour. *Lancet* **341**, 986–8.

World Health Organization (1992). *WHO Laboratory Manual for the Examination of Human Semen and Sperm–Cervical Mucus Interaction,* 3rd edn. Cambridge: Cambridge University Press.

World Health Organization (1999). *WHO Laboratory Manual for the Examination of Human Semen and Sperm-Cervical Mucus Interaction,* 4th edn. Cambridge: Cambridge University Press.

13

Cryopreservation of gametes, ovarian tissue, testicular tissue and embryos; frozen embryo replacement

Introduction

The availability of cryopreservation technology has extended the scope of human assisted conception treatment and made it more convenient for patients. For example, prior freezing of sperm may be the only way in which a couple can have assisted conception treatment if the male partner has to be away at a critical time during the treatment; the frozen sample is thawed and used when required. Donor insemination has become safer because donated semen samples are frozen and quarantined for six months, at the end of which the donor is re-tested for evidence of the human immunodeficiency virus (HIV) infection, or for any of the other screened infections. Good quality embryos frequently remain after transfer of the required number into the woman; these can be frozen and used at a later date, if required, instead of the couple going through another cycle of in vitro fertilization (IVF) treatment. Although more problematic, freezing of oocytes and ovarian tissue is now taking place in research institutions and should hopefully become widely available for clinical use in future. Cryopreservation is an important component of the management strategy for azoospermia using surgical retrieval of sperm directly from the genital tract or from testicular tissue. The conduct of cryopreservation in humans is based on information originally derived from animal work, where sperm cryopreservation for example, has been carried out for several decades for animal breeding. This chapter will consider the principles of cryopreservation followed by a general description of the practical steps. The clinical applications of cryopreservation will also be described. A final section will deal with frozen embryo replacement.

Principles of cryopreservation

Cell injury and death during freezing and thawing is related to the formation of large amounts of ice crystals within the cell. Cryopreservation aims to remove as much of the intracellular water as is compatible with life, before freezing, so as to

Table 13.1. Examples of cryoprotectants

Permeating cryoprotectants
Dimethyl sulphoxide
Glycerol
1-2 Propanediol (propylene glycol)
Methanol
Ethylene glycol
Dimethyl acetamide
Dimethyl formamide
Erythrypiol

Non-permeating cryoprotectants
Sucrose and other sugars
Proteins
Polyvinylpyrrolidone

---

reduce the extent of intracellular ice formation to the point where it ceases to constitute a threat to the viability of the cell. Removal of excessive amounts of water, however, will cause cellular injury and possible death through the effect of the resulting highly concentrated intracellular environment on intracellular components, particularly their membranes. This is called the 'solution' effect. Cryoprotectants are compounds that are used to achieve the required intracellular dehydration. They do so either by entering the cell and displacing the water molecules out of the cell (permeating cryoprotectants) or by remaining largely out of the cell but drawing out the intracellular water by osmosis (non-permeating cryoprotectants). Examples of these compounds are shown in Table 13.1. Usually, combinations of the compounds are used, for example, sucrose and one of the permeating cryoprotectants. Glycerol, dimethyl sulphoxide (DMSO), propanediol and sucrose have been used extensively in human work. Propanediol-sucrose cryoprotectant solutions are used for freezing fertilized eggs at the 2-pronuclei stage and cleavage stage embryos. Glycerol-sucrose cryoprotectant solutions are used for freezing blastocysts. Glycerol is also an important component of sperm freezing solutions. Cryoprotectant solutions contain other compounds that may have protective effects on the cells during freezing and thawing, and they are called extenders. Examples of such compounds include citrate, egg yolk and zwitterionic buffers. The cryoprotectant solution is normally made up by adding measured amounts of these compounds to physiological solutions similar to gamete and embryo culture media. The pH of the cryoprotectant solution is maintained by using HEPES or phosphate buffers. Egg yolk is only used as an extender in sperm cryopreservation media.

Another aspect of cryopreservation that influences the rate of cell survival is the rate of cooling and warming. The optimum cooling rate should be one that allows enough water to leave the cell before intracellular freezing occurs. If freezing occurs before the required amount of water leaves the cell, the degree of intracellular ice crystal formation may become lethal. During thawing there should be a controlled exit of the cryoprotectant from the cell and for the re-entry of the water molecules. If water re-entry into the cell is too rapid it may swell and burst the cell. If the cryoprotectant lingers on longer than it should, it may exert toxic effects on the thawed and now metabolically active cell. Non-permeating cryoprotectants such as sucrose are most useful for their effect in controlling water re-entry into the cell during thawing. There is also a risk of more intracellular ice crystal formation during thawing if the rate of warming is too slow.

Steps in cryopreservation and thawing

The cell or tissue sample (oocyte, embryo or ovarian tissue or testicular tissue) is transferred into the cryoprotectant solution and left there for some minutes depending on the type of cell to be frozen. Protocols for oocyte and embryo freezing usually involve their transfer from weaker cryoprotectant solutions through increasingly stronger solutions. The cell is then transferred into a suitable container such as a plastic straw or glass ampoule ready for freezing (Figure 13.1). The use of glass ampoules is not advisable as they often explode during thawing due to the expansion of the air inside. This may result in loss of the cells frozen inside it. Furthermore flying glass particles constitute a health hazard to laboratory staff.

For sperm freezing, the calculated volume of the cryoprotectant solution is slowly added to the semen sample while swirling the container to ensure proper mixing of the semen with the cryoprotectant solution. This is then allowed to stand on the laboratory bench at room temperature for about 25 minutes to allow enough time for the cryoprotectant to permeate into the sperm. During this period the mixture can be aliquoted into properly labelled polypropylene ampoules or straws ready for freezing (Figure 13.2).

Generally, two methods of freezing are widely used in clinical practice, vapour freezing and the use of programmable freezers. Suspension of the ampoules or straws in liquid nitrogen vapour for about 30 minutes is the more usual method for freezing semen samples. Liquid nitrogen vapour has a temperature of $-85\,°C$; the temperature of the sperm sample when suspended in this vapour, will fall by about $10\,°C$ every minute. Although the vapour freezing process may be complete within 10 minutes it is advisable to leave the ampoules or straws in the vapour for a further 20 minutes to ensure that semen at the core of these containers is well frozen and as close to $-85\,°C$ as possible. At the end of the 30 minute freezing period the

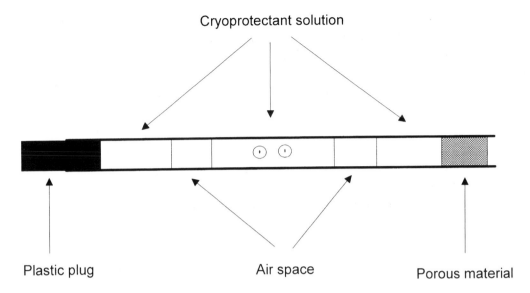

Figure 13.1 Straw containing two cells for cryopreservation. Normally, gentle suction is applied to the end of the straw that is plugged loosely with porous material. The opposite end of the straw is dipped into the cryoprotectant solution and used in aspirating a small volume of fluid before being raised and aspirating some air. The straw is then dipped into the cryoprotectant solution again to aspirate the cells together with some of the solution. Another column of air is drawn in before a final column of cryoprotectant solution. Finally, a plastic plug or other suitable material is used to close that end of the straw.

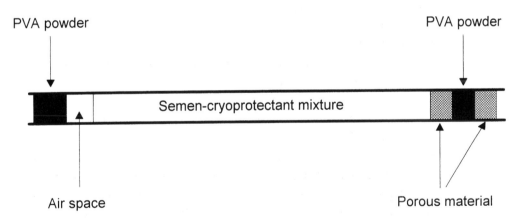

Figure 13.2 Straw filled with semen-cryoprotectant mixture (PVA: polyvinyl alcohol).

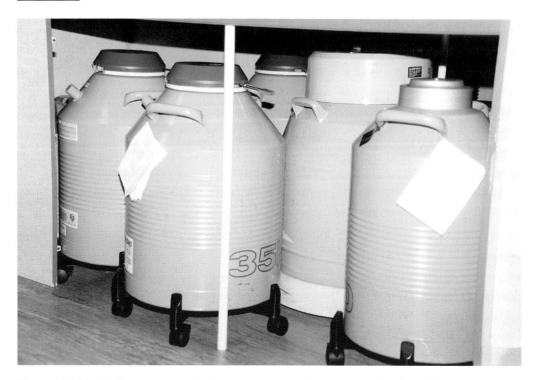

Figure 13.3 Liquid nitrogen dewers for long-term storage of cryopreserved cells and tissue.

ampoules or straws of semen are transferred to storage vats called dewers that contain liquid nitrogen (Figure 13.3). The temperature of liquid nitrogen is −196 °C and the frozen semen containers are stored submerged by the liquid nitrogen. Cells and tissue can be kept in frozen storage for several years without any further deterioration of their quality and survival following thawing.

Embryos, oocytes, ovarian and testicular tissue, and poor quality semen samples can be frozen using a more controlled protocol in an attempt to improve their survival on thawing. This is achieved using computer programmed freezers (Figures 13.4 and 13.5), which slowly lower the temperature of the freezing chambers at set rates until the required temperature is reached when the straws or ampoules are transferred to liquid nitrogen dewers for storage. An example of such a freezing program is presented in Table 13.2.

Relatively rapid thawing procedures are used and involve removal of the straw or ampoule from the dewer and warming it up to 37 °C using various techniques depending on the type of cell(s) or tissue being thawed. Thawing procedures for frozen sperm are shown in Table 13.3. The use of a water bath maintained at 37 °C is usually all that is needed when thawing frozen oocytes, embryos and ovarian and testicular tissues. Following thawing, the cryoprotectant is washed off. For sperm

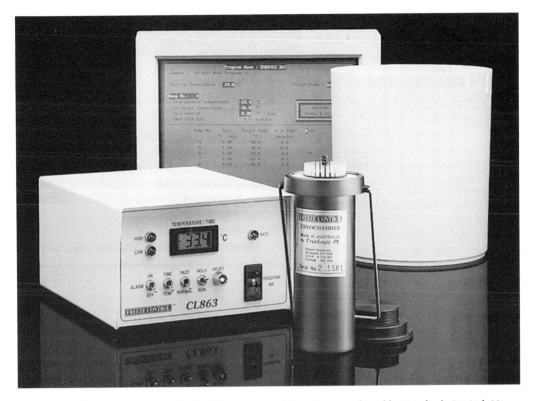

Figure 13.4 The FREEZE CONTROL CL863 programmable system produced by Cryologic Pty Ltd, Mt Waverly, Australia.

this is done by using the sperm preparation techniques described in Chapters 8 and 9. Simple 'washing' with culture medium is adequate for testicular tissue. For oocytes and embryos, serial passage through increasingly weaker cryoprotectant solutions is performed until the final stage which is the transfer into a culture dish containing ordinary gamete or embryo culture medium.

An alternative technique for freezing oocytes and embryos uses a more rapid approach called ultrarapid cooling. Here the temperature of the solution is decreased rapidly, by about 2500°C/minute. This is achieved by plunging the ampoules or straws containing the oocytes or embryos directly into liquid nitrogen from room temperature. The cryoprotectant solution is made up using DMSO and sucrose and their concentration is twice that used in the slow cooling–freezing techniques. This freezing technique is so rapid that it does not allow much time for intracellular ice crystal formation to occur. Even when this occurs it is likely to be in the form of non-lethal small sized crystals.

A variant of ultrarapid cooling is called vitrification on account of the fact that instead of turning into ice crystals the cryoprotectant solution turns into a highly

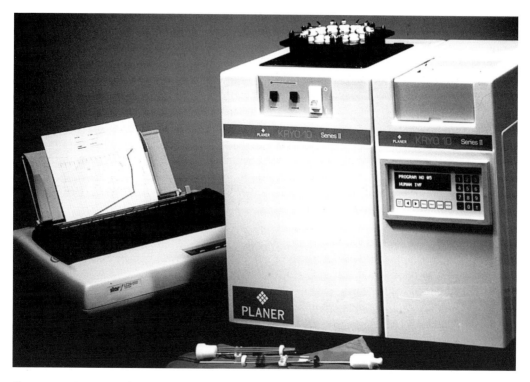

Figure 13.5 Kryo 10 series programmable freezer produced by Planer Products Ltd, Sunbury, UK.

viscous glass-like solid. To achieve this a higher concentration of cryoprotectant than that used for ultrarapid cooling is used in making up the cryoprotectant solution. Glycerol has been used successfully for vitrification.

Intracellular ice crystal formation can still occur during thawing of oocytes and embryos frozen by ultrarapid cooling or vitrification. In order to avoid this, thawing has to be rapid (at least 500 °C/minute) so as to convert the solid frozen water directly into liquid without going through the ice crystal formation stage. Ultrarapid cooling and vitrification have not yet been used in routine clinical practice.

Cryopreservation of sperm

One of the major indications for semen freezing is sperm donation. It allows the maintenance of donor anonymity and is more convenient than using fresh sperm samples. It also allows quarantine of sperm to allow re-testing of donors for HIV and other infections at regular intervals thereafter, most commonly after the first six months. Freezing of sperm is also carried out prior to starting any treatment that may compromise a man's future fertility such as chemotherapy for cancer,

Table 13.2. A slow freezing programme suitable for embryo cryopreservation

1. Cool chamber from 20 °C to −7 °C at the rate of −2 °C/minute
2. Hold chamber temperature at −7 °C for 10 minutes to allow the controlled induction of ice formation (called seeding) in the straw or ampoule
3. Cool chamber from −7 °C to −30 °C at the rate of −0.8 °C/minute
4. Hold chamber temperature at −30 °C for 10 minutes
5. Cool chamber from −30 °C to −150 °C at the rate of −50 °C/minute*

Notes:

*At the end of this programme remove the straws or ampoules from the freezer and transfer immediately into storage dewer

Table 13.3. Human sperm thawing protocols

- Room temperature for 10 minutes and 37 °C for 10 minutes
- Ice water for 10 minutes and 37 °C for 10 minutes
- 35 °C water bath for 12 seconds and 37 °C for 10 minutes
- Rubbing the straws between the fingers
- Holding the straws or ampoules in the hand (not advised as it may cause burns)
- 37 °C water bath until sample is thawed

radiotherapy of the testes and adjoining areas for testicular tumours or surgical removal of testicular tumours. Some men may elect to have their sperm frozen prior to undergoing vasectomy. This is in the event that their circumstances change in future and they wish to have more children. Men with worsening sperm counts and other seminal profiles can have sperm samples frozen as some of these men eventually become azoospermic. As introduced earlier on in this chapter another indication for sperm freezing is the absentee partner. Such partners may have to be away on business or at work at the time when the insemination or IVF treatment is to take place. Other examples include partners who are in prison. Semen collected from men who have ejaculatory dysfunction is normally frozen for potential use in future. The same also applies to sperm that is retrieved surgically from men with azoospermia (see Chapter 10).

Sperm survival is not invariable following freeze–thawing. However, enough sperm usually survive to allow fertility treatment to proceed as planned. Poor quality sperm samples tend to have poor survival. This does not mean that such samples should not be frozen provided further samples are not of better quality. With the availability of intracytoplasmic sperm injection (ICSI) only few live sperm are required for injection into all retrieved eggs (usually not more than 20) that are suitable. Most laboratories will carry out a test thaw on every batch of frozen semen within 24 hours of the freezing procedure. One of the ampoules or straws is removed from the liquid nitrogen dewer, thawed and analysed. The sperm survival rate and post-thaw motility characteristics are documented.

Donor sperm banks adopt more stringent criteria; for example many banks will only accept donors if the sperm survival is at least 50%. There may be occasions when less stringent criteria are used, especially if the donor comes from an under-represented ethnic group or there is a scarcity of more suitable donors.

Cryopreservation of testicular tissue

Testicular tissue can be surgically obtained from men with azoospermia using a number of techniques that have been described in Chapter 10. Following process-ing, sperm can be identified and extracted from the tissue samples for injection into oocytes; several thousand pregnancies and children have resulted from this proce-dure (see Chapter 9). Cryopreservation technology has removed some of the uncer-tainty regarding the availability of viable sperm on the day of oocyte retrieval. Without cryopreservation the treatment strategy will have to take into considera-tion the chance that viable sperm may not be found if testicular tissue retrieval is performed on the same day for which oocyte retrieval is planned. The risk of unsuc-cessful sperm retrieval is higher in men with secretory azoospermia than in those with obstructive azoospermia. If sperm retrieval is unsuccessful on the planned day for oocyte retrieval it means that either the oocyte retrieval has to be cancelled thereby losing all the money spent up to that point in the treatment or donor sperm used in fertilizing the oocytes following retrieval. These undesirable options can be largely avoided by carrying out testicular sperm retrieval before commencing ovarian stimulation. If sperm is retrieved they are cryopreserved. Alternatively, the testicular tissue is cryopreserved once it is demonstrated to contain viable sperm. A test thaw is performed the next day to ascertain the possibility of extracting viable sperm from the thawed testicular tissue sample. When it is impossible to obtain sperm the couple will have enough time to decide on options available to them including the use of donor sperm and receive appropriate counselling before com-mencing on ovarian stimulation.

Cryopreservation of oocytes

Cryopreservation of oocytes has not been very successful so far due to the poor sur-vival of frozen oocytes following thawing. The exact reason for this is unknown but cold temperature is known to disorganize the spindle fibre of the oocyte. This is the structure that is formed during cell division and ensures the orderly separation of chromosomes and their segregation into the resulting daughter cells. The ideal candidate for oocyte cryopreservation is the young unmarried girl who develops a cancer and has to have the potentially castrating treatments of chemotherapy, pelvic irradiation (radiotherapy) or surgical removal of the ovaries. Such patients, time permitting, can have ovarian stimulation and oocyte retrieval followed by cryopreservation of the oocytes. If the patient survives the cancer and wishes to become pregnant in future the oocytes can be thawed and fertilized using ICSI. The use of ICSI instead of conventional IVF to procure fertilization is thought prudent because the freeze–thaw process may have altered some of the constituents of the zona pellucida and cell membrane creating uncertainty about the ability of the sperm to penetrate those layers and fuse with the oocyte. As shown in Chapter 9, ICSI bypasses all these barriers and deposits the sperm within the cytoplasm of the oocyte. The appropriate number of resulting embryos are subsequently transferred into the uterus. In such cases development of the uterine endometrium is stimulated and maintained using oestrogen tablets and progesterone pessaries as described in a later section for frozen embryo replacement.

Cryopreservation of ovarian tissue

It may at times be inadvisable for the patient described above to undergo ovarian stimulation as this may take up to six weeks to complete and the use of ovarian stimulants may worsen the prognosis of the disease. In such instances ovarian tissue is obtained by biopsy, cut into small portions and frozen. Animal work has shown that successful ovarian follicular development and ovulation can occur when these pieces of ovarian tissue are thawed and grafted back to the animal from which it was taken. It is also possible to microdissect thawed pieces of ovarian tissue to release the immature oocytes. These are then cultured in the laboratory until they are mature. They are then fertilized using ICSI. These are still research procedures but there is an expectation that such techniques will become available for clinical use in future (Meniru & Craft, 1997a,b). Dr. Roger Gosden has been a pioneer in this field and the advanced reader is referred to publications (e.g. Newton et al., 1996) emanating from his unit for further information.

Cryopreservation of embryos

Contemporary ovarian stimulation protocols for IVF aim at the production of many oocytes as a way of assuring the generation of enough good quality embryos for transfer. More often than not good quality embryos still remain after transfer of the required number of embryos into the woman and these can be frozen. Survival of frozen embryos after thawing using good techniques is usually above 70% and pregnancy rates following frozen embryo transfers can reach 30% or more. Embryo cryopreservation is therefore a viable component of assisted conception treatment. There are other indications for embryo cryopreservation. This includes situations where there is a high risk of a woman having severe ovarian hyperstimulation syndrome (OHSS); all embryos are frozen and the severe OHSS managed appropriately using drugs, some of which would not have been utilized for fear of teratogenicity if the woman had embryo transfer. When the woman is fully recovered, frozen embryo transfer is carried out (as will be described in the following section). The overwhelming presence of poor prognostic factors in an index IVF treatment cycle may be a reason for freezing all embryos generated. Such factors include intermittent bleeding during the period of ovarian stimulation, poor endometrial development and receptivity as can be deduced using ultrasound scanning and doppler studies. The discovery of uterine pathology during the treatment such as uterine polyps or large, cavity distorting leiomyoma is another indication for embryo cryostorage pending surgical correction of these structural anomalies. All embryos can be frozen and stored following biopsy for pre-implantation genetic diagnosis (PGD) until the results become available. Normally, PGD is arranged such that results become available within 24 hours allowing disease-free embryos to be transferred during that same treatment cycle. Embryos can also be frozen in oocyte or embryo donation cycles to allow greater flexibility in scheduling embryo transfers to the recipient. It can also be used to quarantine these embryos until the donor is re-tested and found disease-free after six months. Embryos can be frozen at the pronuclear, cleavage or blastocyst stage of development but the cryoprotectant used may vary depending on the stage of embryo development at the time of freezing.

Frozen embryo transfer

Frozen human embryos have now been used for treating infertile couples for many years and have resulted in the birth of several thousand healthy babies. Following thawing, these embryos are replaced in the uterus at the correct time in relation to ovulation and the thickness of the endometrium. The frozen embryo replacement cycle is relatively non-invasive compared to an egg collection cycle. The embryos can be replaced either in a natural cycle or in a hormone-controlled cycle. In a controlled cycle a gonadotrophin releasing hormone agonist, such as Zoladex, Prostap, Nafarelin, Buserelin or Lupron is first administered to suppress the pituitary gland (see Chapter 8). Oestrogen tablets, such as Progynova, are administered daily to prepare the endometrium for implantation as an alternative to the natural changes occurring in the endometrium in a spontaneous ovulatory cycle.

The development of the endometrium is monitored by ultrasound scanning; approximately four episodes of scanning will be required, although it can be less (see Appendix 13.1). Either when ovulation has occurred, or when the endometrium is thick enough (ideally 9 mm or more), the embryos can be thawed for replacement. The embryos will be thawed so that the developmental stage of the embryos corresponds to the replacement cycle day. The exact timing will depend upon the stage at which the embryos were frozen.

Not all embryos survive the freezing, storage and thawing process. On the morning of the embryo transfer, the embryos are assessed to see if they are suitable for transfer. If they are, then the embryo transfer can proceed. For this procedure a fine catheter is passed through the cervix and the embryos are injected high into the uterus in a minute amount of culture medium.

Progesterone preparations, such as Cyclogest, are provided for daily or twice daily insertion into the rectum or vagina from where it is absorbed into the blood circulation to support the endometrium. A pregnancy test is carried out with a blood sample that is withdrawn 12 days after the embryo transfer. The success rate using frozen thawed embryos is between 10 and 30% or more, depending on the individual patient's particular situation and the experience of that IVF unit. A sample treatment schedule/instruction sheet for patients undergoing frozen embryo replacement treatment is given in Appendix 13.1.

Conclusion

Cryopreservation of gametes and embryos is now an established component of assisted conception treatment. It has brought far reaching changes to the management of patients including making treatment safer by the quarantine of donated gametes and embryos, more flexibility and convenience. Improvement in cryosurvival is still needed especially for frozen–thawed oocytes. This will make it easier to avoid current moral and legal problems relating to long-term storage of embryos or their disposal. Setting up donor oocyte banks will also become more feasible.

Appendix 13.1. Frozen embryo replacement: treatment schedule and instructions

Treatment cycle day	Day/date	Comments/instruction
0 minus		• You may be given tablets to readjust your menstrual cycle. This will not be necessary for every patient
0 minus		• GnRHa (e.g. Zoladex, Nafarelin or Buserelin) administration starts
0 minus		• Baseline ULTRASOUND SCAN (Time $=\ldots$)
		• Blood tests, final instructions, consents etc
1		• 2 mg tablet of Progynova taken twice a day
2		• 2 mg tablet of Progynova taken twice a day

Appendix 13.1. (*cont.*)

Treatment cycle day	Day/date	Comments/instruction
3		• 2 mg tablet of Progynova taken twice a day
4		• 2 mg tablet of Progynova taken twice a day
5		• 2 mg tablet of Progynova taken twice a day
6		• 2 mg tablet of Progynova taken twice a day
7		• 2 mg tablet of Progynova taken twice a day
8		• 2 mg tablet of Progynova taken THREE TIMES a day
9		• 2 mg tablet of Progynova taken THREE TIMES a day
10		• 2 mg tablet of Progynova taken THREE TIMES a day
11		• 2 mg tablet of Progynova taken THREE TIMES a day
12		• 2 mg tablet of Progynova taken THREE TIMES a day
13		• 2 mg tablet of Progynova taken THREE TIMES a day
14		• 2 mg tablet of Progynova taken THREE TIMES a day
		• Stop using Nafarelin or Buserelin nasal spray
		• ULTRASOUND SCAN (Time = ...)
15		• 2 mg tablet of Progynova taken THREE TIMES a day
		• 400 mg Cyclogest pessary inserted twice a day
16		• 2 mg tablet of Progynova taken THREE TIMES a day
		• 400 mg Cyclogest pessary inserted twice a day
17		• 2 mg tablet of Progynova taken THREE TIMES a day
		• 400 mg Cyclogest pessary inserted twice a day
		• *Insert Cyclogest pessaries into the rectum this morning*
		• Embryo transfer should normally take place today
		• Time ...
From Day 18 until pregnancy test Two weeks after embryo transfer		• 2 mg tablet of Progynova taken THREE TIMES a day
		• 400 mg Cyclogest pessary inserted twice a day
		• Come for a blood test to find out if you are pregnant
		• Go home after the blood sample is taken. Your doctor will ring you back with the results that same day
		• If your menses start before this date it is most likely that you are NOT pregnant. Call us. If after speaking with you we are sure you are having your periods we will instruct you to stop using Progynova and Cyclogest
		• If the pregnancy test result shows that you are pregnant, you will need to continue with Progynova tablets (2 mg tablet of Progynova taken THREE TIMES a day) and Cyclogest pessaries (400 mg twice daily) until you are 12 weeks pregnant

Wishing you the best of luck in your treatment.

BIBLIOGRAPHY

Audrins, P., Holden, C. A., McLachlan, R. I. & Kovacs, G. (1999). Semen storage for special purposes at Monash IVF from 1977 to 1997. *Fertility and Sterility* **72**, 179–81.

Dale, B. & Elder, K. (1997). *In vitro fertilization.* Cambridge: Cambridge University Press.

Ferraretti, A. P., Gianaroli, L., Magli, C. et al. (1999). Elective cryopreservation of all pronucleate embryos in women at risk of ovarian hyperstimulation syndrome: efficiency and safety. *Human Reproduction* **14**, 1457–60.

Hong, S. W., Chung, H. M., Lim, J. M. et al. (1999). Improved human oocyte development after vitrification: a comparison of thawing methods. *Fertility and Sterility* **72**, 142–6.

Meniru, G. I. & Craft, I. L. (1997a). Assisted conception options for patients with good-prognosis cervical cancer. *Lancet* **349**, 542.

Meniru, G. I. & Craft, I. L. (1997b). In-vitro fertilization and embryo cryopreservation prior to hysterectomy for cervical cancer. *International Journal of Gynecology and Obstetrics* **56**, 69–70.

Newton, H., Aubard, Y., Rutherford, A. et al. (1996). Low temperature storage and grafting of human ovarian tissue. *Human Reproduction* **11**, 1487–91.

Quinn, P. (1995). Cryopreservation of embryos and oocytes. In *Infertility Evaluation and Treatment*, ed. W. R. Keye, R. J. Chang, R. W. Rebar & M. R. Soules, pp. 821–40. Philadelphia: W. B. Saunders and Co.

Trad, F. S., Toner, M. & Biggers, J. D. (1999). Effects of cryoprotectants and ice-seeding temperature on intracellular freezing and survival of human oocytes. *Human Reproduction* **14**, 1569–77.

Trounson, A. & Mohr, L. (1983). Human pregnancy following cryopreservation, thawing and transfer of an eight-cell embryo. *Nature* **305**, 707–9.

Tucker, M., Wright, G., Morton, P. et al. (1996). Preliminary experience with human oocyte cryopreservation using 1,2-propanediol and sucrose. *Human Reproduction* **11**, 1513–15.

14

Assisted hatching

Introduction

Several factors affect the chances of conception following treatment with conventional in vitro fertilization (IVF) or any of its variants. However, while the negative influence of factors such as increasing age of the female is known, many others still remain unknown. The normal process of human embryo hatching seems to be another one of those factors. The embryo must 'hatch' through the zona pellucida before it can implant. Although the exact mechanisms are not fully understood, this may involve the production of compounds, called lysins, by the embryo and/or endometrium that dissolve the zona pellucida thereby reducing its thickness. The blastocyst then expands and contracts repeatedly leading to further thinning and eventual rupture of the zona pellucida. It is possible that a defective hatching process is a cause of failed implantation in some women who have IVF treatment. The most common hypothesis to explain this phenomenon is that of abnormal zona hardening. Following fusion of the sperm with the oolemma of the oocyte the chemical constitution of the zona pellucida changes somewhat and in so doing prevents penetration by more spermatozoa. The process of excess zona hardening can occur spontaneously and to a greater degree following gonadotrophin therapy and in vitro culture. Another reason for non-hatching of the cleaving embryo can be the presence of an unduly thick zona pellucida. Observations on the pattern of hatching of animal and human embryos generated from microassisted fertilization (see Chapter 9) led the pioneer worker Dr. Jacques Cohen and his colleagues to propose that the artificial creation of an opening in the zona pellucida could lead to improved hatching rates for embryos resulting in higher implantation and pregnancy rates. The procedure of 'assisted hatching' (Cohen, 1992) has now been studied further by many research groups to determine its use as an adjunct assisted conception treatment method and the patient groups who may benefit from its performance.

Table 14.1. Indications for assisted hatching

Thick zona pellucida
Older age (>38 years)
Patients with elevated FSH levels
Repeated unsuccessful treatment with IVF or its variants
Embryos generated from in vitro matured oocytes

Notes:
FSH: follicle stimulating hormone; IVF: in vitro fertilization.

Patient selection

While some workers have applied assisted hatching to all patients in their series (Hu et al., 1996), others have proposed a more selective approach in the belief that the natural hatching process may not be dysfunctional in all patients who have IVF treatment. The main indications that have been applied in the published literature can be found in Table 14.1. Thickness of the zona pellucida has been implicated as a cause for defective hatching by Cohen et al. (1992). Their studies strongly suggest that embryos whose zonae were thicker than 15 μm were less likely to implant than those with thinner zonae or those with zonae that had been drilled. Further retrospective analysis of their data and prospective evaluation of patient groups have also identified older women and females with elevated follicle stimulating hormone (FSH) levels as benefiting from assisted hatching (Cohen, 1995). The thickness of the zona pellucida does not seem to correlate with the age of the woman; zona hardening seems to be the main reason for defective embryo hatching in older women and those with elevated FSH levels. Repeated failure to become pregnant following IVF treatment is obviously multifactorial but assisted hatching seems to be successful when applied in subsequent treatment cycles (Schoolcraft et al., 1994; Antinori et al., 1996b). Finally, an increasing number of reports on in vitro culture of immature oocytes are now being published. Such oocytes are usually inseminated using intracytoplasmic sperm injection (see Chapter 9) and assisted hatching performed on the resulting embryos before they are transferred into the uterus. Assisted hatching in such cases is based on the theoretical assumption that prolonged in vitro culture required for maturation of the oocyte will cause hardening of the zona pellucida.

Overview of techniques

Micromanipulation of the embryo for assisted hatching is usually performed on Day 3 following oocyte retrieval. At this stage the embryo contains six or more cells.

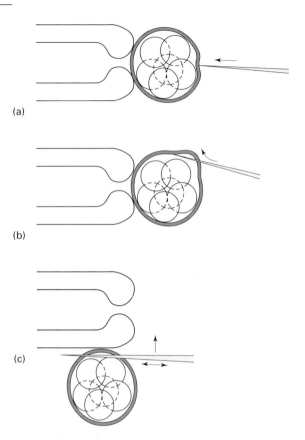

(a)

(b)

(c)

Figure 14.1 Assisted hatching using partial zona dissection: (a) the zona pellucida is pierced with a microneedle at a point overlying the indentation between two adjacent blastomeres; (b) the microneedle is manoeuvred forwards and upwards to pierce the zona pellucida again at some distance away from the original point of entry; (c) the suction grip of the holding pipette on the embryo is discontinued so that the pipette can be moved and used in rubbing against the part of the zona pellucida that is lying between it and the microneedle to slit open that part of the zona pellucida.

The reason for delaying the procedure until the third day is that intercellular connections start to form at this stage thereby preventing loss of the blastomeres (embryo cells) following opening of the zona pellucida. Techniques that do not involve creating holes in the zona pellucida can be performed on Day 2 and the embryos transferred into the uterus on that same day. Some workers have, however, performed zona drilling on the Day 2 human embryo (Antinori et al., 1996b).

Partial zona dissection (PZD)

This technique has already been mentioned in Chapter 9. In fact, early observations by Cohen and colleagues were made on patients who had PZD to improve the

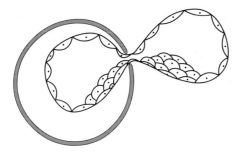

Figure 14.2 Schematic representation of an embryo in the process of hatching through a hole made in the zona pellucida. The hatching embryo may become trapped if the hole is not large enough, creating a figure-of-eight appearance.

chances of fertilization because of male factor infertility. PZD is performed with a microneedle or microblade which is used to create a slit of varying length in the zona pellucida (Figure 14.1). The instruments are mounted on a micromanipulation microscope as described in Chapter 9. The size of the hole made by PZD is critical. Embryo hatching though a narrow hole often fails due to inability of the whole of the embryo to negotiate the narrow passage. In fact a figure-of-eight embryo shape is often described in such situations (Figure 14.2) and is formed by part of the embryo lying outside the zona pellucida but retaining contact, through the narrow hole in the zona pellucida, with the rest of the embryo that is trapped within the enclosure formed by the zona pellucida. There is also a possibility of damage to the embryonic cells with rearrangement of their spatial relationship to each other. One consequence of this may be an increased incidence of monozygotic twinning after PZD (Hershlag et al., 1999).

Zona drilling

A large proportion of studies on assisted hatching have been carried out using acidified Tyrode's solution to bring about thinning of the zona pellucida (Figure 14.3). The constituents of this solution are shown in Table 14.2. Equally good zona thinning results can be obtained by using culture medium that has been acidified (pH 2.4) by the addition of hydrochloric acid. Again a microscope with a micromanipulation set-up is used. The pipette on the left side is the holding pipette and stabilizes the embryo while the pipette on the right side is loaded with acidified Tyrode's solution and brought close to the side of the embryo. Care is taken to position the tip of the right micropipette beside the zona pellucida such that it is overlying the space between two blastomeres rather than lying directly over a blastomere. A controlled flow of Tyrode's solution is directed at the zona pellucida and its dissolution carefully monitored. When most of the intervening layers of the zona

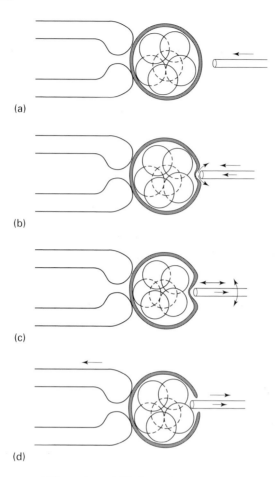

(a)

(b)

(c)

(d)

Figure 14.3 Zona drilling using acidified Tyrode's solution: (a) the embryo is held in position with the holding pipette; (b) a controlled flow of pre-loaded acidified Tyrode's solution is directed at the part of the zona pellucida that overlies the indentation between two adjacent blastomeres; (c) the flow of acidified Tyrode's solution is stopped when most of the layers of the zona pellucida dissolve. The micropipette is then used in pushing through the remaining layers and widening the hole made in the zona pellucida; (d) the micropipette and holding pipette are withdrawn.

pellucida have dissolved, the flow of the solution is stopped and the pipette tip used to push through the final layers to complete breaching of the zona pellucida. The embryo is then washed with fresh culture medium and transferred to a dish of fresh culture medium.

Lasers

The use of lasers allows a greater degree of control and more precision during assisted hatching. Lasers can be used in thinning the zona pellucida (Antinori et al.,

Table 14.2. Composition of acidified Tyrode's solution

Component	Weight (grams)
NaCl	8.0
KCl	0.2
$CaCl_2.2H_2O$	0.2
$MgCl_2.6H_2O$	0.1
$NaH_2PO_4.H_2O$	0.05
Glucose	1.0
Polyvinylpyrrolidone	4.0

Notes:
Add these compounds to one litre of water which should be sterile and of culture grade quality.
Finally add hydrochloric acid to the solution until the pH reaches 2.3–2.5.
Source: Adapted from Cohen (1992).

Table 14.3. Laser systems that have been used for assisted hatching

Argon fluoride laser at 193 nm
Erbium:YAG laser at 2940 nm
PALM UV laser at 337 nm
Neodymium:YAG laser at 1064 nm
Xenon chloride excimer laser at 308 nm
Krypton fluoride at 248 nm
Diode laser at 1.48 μm

Source: References in Antinori et al. (1996a,b).

1996a) or creating a full thickness breach (Antinori et al., 1996b). A number of laser systems have now been reported on (Table 14.3), and there is continuing evaluation to determine the most effective and least hazardous of these systems. Laser thinning of the zona pellucida has been proposed as being more natural than laser drilling because it allows blastocyst expansion and hatching that is more analogous to what is found in nature. Furthermore, since no hole is made in the zona pellucida loss of blastomeres or the whole of the embryo is prevented and no toxic chemicals, bacteria or white blood cells are allowed to come into contact with the embryo (Antinori et al., 1996a). Lasers can be used in the 'contact' mode, in which case the laser fibre is placed against the zona pellucida before application of the laser beam. The laser fibre should be disposable or is capable of being sterilized before being used on another patient's embryos. 'Non-contact' laser delivery systems (Antinori et al., 1996b) have also been described and have become more popular as they are quite easy to use. Most importantly none of the equipment comes into contact with the embryo or culture medium thereby avoiding problems of cross-contamination.

Clinical management

Patients undergoing assisted hatching are usually administered prophylactic antibiotics and steroids. The use of broad spectrum antibiotics is believed to eradicate any micro-organisms that may be introduced into the uterine cavity during embryo replacement. Administration of corticosteroids such as prednisolone is expected to modify the patient's immune response such that the number of white blood cells in the uterine cavity is decreased. Both measures should decrease the chances of the embryo being attacked through the breach in the zona pellucida. The utility of these interventions is, however, not clear so they have to be regarded as being empirical for the time being.

Results of assisted hatching

Cohen (1995) reviewed the combined results of three randomized prospective trials, involving 330 patients, that were conducted at the Center for Reproductive Medicine and Infertility, New York Hospital-Cornell Medical Center. The clinical pregnancy rate (52% or 85/164) and the implantation rate (27% or 147/555) following zona drilling was significantly higher than the respective rates obtained in the control group (37%, or 62/166, and 19%, or 104/555). Several other reports have confirmed the improved treatment outcome following assisted hatching (Schoolcraft et al., 1995) but there are also studies that do not demonstrate any difference in outcome (Stein et al., 1995; Bider et al., 1997; Lanzendorf et al., 1998; Edirisinghe et al., 1999). The reasons for these are not readily obvious but may reflect differing operator skill, study populations and methodologies.

Conclusion

Assisted hatching is one of several interventions that have been applied during IVF treatment in an attempt to boost pregnancy rates. Further study using standardized techniques and well-defined study populations will allow a more confident appraisal of the results. The advent of laser zona drilling will avoid the possible embryo toxicity experienced by some workers using acidified Tyrode's solution. Lasers will also permit more precise and reproducible openings to be made in the zona pellucida. It will be easier to describe the parameters of such openings including their relationship to various landmarks in the embryo. One possible benefit of such mapping exercises is that drilling at a particular pole of the embryo may be found to give the best results. Another issue that needs to be settled relates to whether all patients should have zona micromanipulation for assisted hatching or if only a well-selected group should have it performed on their embryos. Finally, this intervention increases the risk of monozygotic twinning which is fascinating biologically but also increases the risk to the pregnancy.

BIBLIOGRAPHY

Antinori, S., Panci, C., Selman, H. A. et al. (1996a). Zona thinning with the use of laser: a new approach to assisted hatching in humans. *Human Reproduction* **11**, 590–4.

Antinori, S., Selman, H. A., Caffa, B. et al. (1996b). Zona opening of human embryos using a non-contact UV laser for assisted hatching in patients with poor prognosis of pregnancy. *Human Reproduction* **11**, 2488–92.

Bider, D., Livshits, A., Yonish, M. et al. (1997). Assisted hatching by zona drilling of human embryos in women of advanced age. *Human Reproduction* **12**, 317–20.

Cohen, J. (1992). Zona pellucida micromanipulation and consequences for embryonic development and implantation. In *Micromanipulation of Human Gametes and Embryos*, ed. J. Cohen, H. E. Malter, B. E. Talansky & J. Grifo, pp. 191–222. New York: Raven Press.

Cohen, J. (1995). Micromanipulation of human gametes, zygotes, and embryos. In *Infertility Evaluation and Treatment*, ed. W. R. Keye, R. J. Chang, R. W. Rebar & M. R. Soules, pp. 841–58. Philadelphia: W. B. Saunders Company.

Cohen, J., Elsner, C., Kort, H. et al. (1990). Impairment of the hatching process following IVF in the human and improvement of implantation by assisting hatching using micromanipulation. *Human Reproduction* **5**, 7–13.

Cohen, J., Alikani, M., Trowbridge, J. & Rosenwaks, Z. (1992). Implantation enhancement by selective assisted hatching using zona drilling of human embryos with poor prognosis. *Human Reproduction* **7**, 685–91.

Cohen, J., Malter, H. E., Talansky, B. E. & Grifo, J. (1992). *Micromanipulation of Human Gametes and Embryos*. New York: Raven Press.

Edirisinghe, W. R., Ahnonkitpanit, V., Promvienghchai, S. et al. (1999). A study failing to determine significant benefits from assisted hatching: patients selected for advanced age, zonal thickness of embryos, and previous failed attempts. *Journal of Assisted Reproduction and Genetics* **16**, 294–301.

Hershlag, A., Paine, T., Cooper, G. W. et al. (1999). Monozygotic twinning associated with mechanical assisted hatching. *Fertility and Sterility* **71**, 144–6.

Hu, Y., Hoffman, D. I., Maxson, W. S. & Ory, S. J. (1996). Clinical application of nonselective assisted hatching of human embryos. *Fertility and Sterility* **66**, 991–4.

Khalifa, E., Tuker, M. J. & Hunt, P. (1992). Cruciate thinning of the zona pellucida for more successful enhancement of blastocyst hatching in the mouse. *Human Reproduction* **7**, 532–6.

Lanzendorf, S. E., Nehchiri, F., Mayer, J. F. et al. (1998). A prospective, randomized, double blind study for the evaluation of assisted hatching in patients with advanced maternal age. *Human Reproduction* **13**, 409–13.

Malter, H. E. & Cohen, J. (1989). Blastocyst formation and hatching *in vitro* following zona drilling of mouse and human embryos. *Gamete Research* **24**, 67–80.

Neev, J., Gonzalez, A., Licciardi, F. et al. (1993). Opening of the mouse zona pellucida by laser without a micromanipulator. *Human Reproduction* **8**, 939–44.

Obruca, A., Strohmer, H., Sakkas, D. et al. (1994). Use of lasers in assisted fertilization and hatching. *Human Reproduction* **9**, 1723–6.

Schoolcraft, W., Schlenker, T., Gee, M. et al. (1994). Assisted hatching in the treatment of poor prognosis *in vitro* fertilization candidates. *Fertility and Sterility* **62**, 551–4.

Schoolcraft, W. B., Schlenker, T., Jones, G. S. & Jones, H. W. Jr. (1995). In vitro fertilization in women age 40 and older: the impact of assisted hatching. *Journal of Assisted Reproduction and Genetics* **12**, 581–4.

Stein, A., Rufas, O., Amit, S. et al. (1995). Assisted hatching by partial zona dissection of human pre-embryos in patients with recurrent implantation failure after *in vitro* fertilization. *Fertility and Sterility* **63**, 834–41.

Strohmer, H. & Feichtinger, W. (1992). Successful clinical application of laser for micromanipulation in an in vitro fertilization program. *Fertility and Sterility* **58**, 212–14.

Tadir, Y., Neev, J., Ho, P. & Berns, M. W. (1993). Laser for gamete micromanipulation: basic concepts. *Journal of Assisted Reproduction and Genetics* **10**, 121–5.

Tucker, M. J., Cohen, J., Massey, J. B. et al. (1991). Partial dissection of the zona pellucida of frozen–thawed human embryos may enhance blastocyst hatching, implantation and pregnancy rates. *American Journal of Obstetrics and Gynecology* **165**, 341–5.

15

Preimplantation diagnosis of genetic disease

Introduction

Genetic disorders are not uncommon, affecting 1–3% of individuals at birth. Some are incompatible with life, leading to death in utero or at some stage (days to years) after birth. Two approaches have been adopted towards the management of these illnesses namely prevention and treatment. Curative treatment has so far been impossible but supportive treatment may improve quality of life and life expectancy in some cases. A number of preventive measures are possible depending on the circumstances. A few individuals may choose the option of not getting married at all but many couples may already be married by the time the disorder is discovered in one of the partners, their parents, children or siblings. Another preventive measure is to choose a partner whose genetic constitution guarantees that offspring from the union will not manifest the clinical effects of the disease although they may be carriers, for example sickle cell anaemia and thalassaemia. These are autosomal recessive diseases and will usually manifest clinically only in the homozygous condition. Other couples have chosen not to have children especially when the problem is invariably fatal and manifests even in the heterozygous state. One other option is the use of donor gametes, in place of one or both partner's gametes, to generate embryos that are free of the disease in question, using artificial insemination or in vitro fertilization (IVF). Donor embryos can also be used in cases where both donor sperm and oocytes are required.

Genetic diagnostic tests can be carried out using placental tissue obtained through chorionic villus sampling in early pregnancy. Alternatively desquamated fetal cells can be obtained from amniotic fluid using amniocentesis in the midtrimester. Patients then have the option of having an affected pregnancy terminated or to continue with the pregnancy. Ultrasound scanning in pregnancy can also reveal structural indications of genetic disease. Termination of pregnancy may not be acceptable to everyone for religious, moral and emotional reasons. The relatively recent advent of preimplantation genetic diagnosis (PGD) has now provided another and probably more acceptable option for affected couples. This

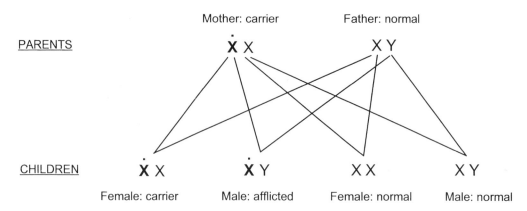

Figure 15.1 The risk of passing on X-linked genetic disease to progeny: the mother is a carrier while the father has normal sex chromosomes.

chapter assumes the reader has a basic knowledge of genetics and associated techniques.

Diseases to screen

In PGD, the genetic defect is either diagnosed or, in the case of sex linked diseases, the sex of the embryos determined, thereby allowing for the transfer of only non-affected or carrier embryos into the uterus. Sexing of embryos makes it possible for couples who have one of 300 or more X-linked recessive diseases that have been reported in the literature, to have children who are free of the disease. Usually the female only manifests the effects of the genetic disorder when both X chromosomes carry similar gene defects. As the male only has one X chromosome the disease manifests whenever the genetic defect is present in that X chromosome. If only female embryos are transferred it means the couple can have female children although 50% of them may be carriers of the genetic disease (Figure 15.1). Most couples are likely to accept this rather than face a childless future. It has now been possible to screen directly for Duchenne muscular dystrophy (Lee et al., 1998), Lesch–Nyhan syndrome and an increasing number of X-linked disorders. Such progress in PGD is welcome as it improves the efficiency of the process; not all male embryos then need to be discarded since 50% of them would have inherited the unaffected X chromosome from the mother (Figure 15.1). Furthermore, it will be possible to be more selective of female embryos that are transferred given that 50% of them would have inherited the normal X chromosome from the mother in addition to the normal paternally derived X chromosome.

PGD may be useful for couples where the male partner has an X-linked recessive disorder, and they do not wish to have children who are carriers. None of their male

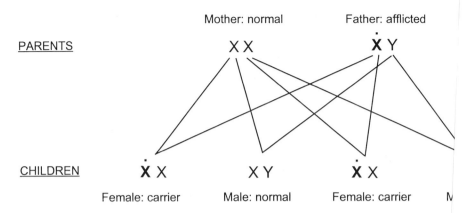

Figure 15.2 The risk of passing on X-linked genetic disease to progeny: the mother is nor~
father has X-linked disease.

progeny will have the disease or be carriers but all female children w~
(Figure 15.2). Sexing of the embryos and transfer of only male embryo~ ......
the avoidance of carrier status in their children and interrupt the potential transfer
of disease to future generations.

PGD of many non-sex linked single gene defects, for example, sickle cell
anaemia, Tay–Sachs disease, haemophilia and cystic fibrosis is now possible
(Verlinsky et al., 1997; Rechitsky et al., 1999). Xu et al. (1999) recently reported on
the birth of unaffected twins following PGD for sickle cell anaemia. This seems to
have been the first of such reports in the scientific literature. Techniques for the
detection of other genetic aberrations, including defects in chromosomal number
and translocations have already been developed and are in routine use (Bahce et al.,
1999; Gianaroli et al., 1999; Staessen et al., 1999).

Generation of embryos for genetic diagnosis

Theoretical considerations

Embryos for PGD can either be recovered from the female genital tract or generated through IVF or intracytoplasmic sperm injection (ICSI). Embryo recovery
from the female genital is least invasively achieved by uterine lavage four to five days
following ovulation and timed intercourse. That is when the embryo is supposed
to enter the uterine cavity following fertilization and early embryonic development
within the fallopian tube. Uterine lavage can be carried out in a natural cycle following mono-ovulation and the generation of a single embryo. Alternatively, to
increase the number of embryos, the woman is administered gonadotrophin injections in the follicular phase of her menstrual cycle to stimulate the production and

ovulation of many oocytes. Timed sexual intercourse or intrauterine insemination is then performed.

Uterine lavage suffers from a number of potential drawbacks. The day of embryo entry into the uterine cavity may vary amongst women thus leading to failed embryo recovery if uterine lavage is performed prior to the embryo(s) reaching the uterine cavity. There is also a possibility that some or all embryos would have implanted by the time the lavage is carried out leading to high order multiple pregnancy. The manipulations required for the performance of uterine lavage may introduce infection leading to endometritis and/or pelvic infection. There is a risk of flushing embryos back into the fallopian tube leading to ectopic pregnancy. Finally, any genetically affected embryo that is not flushed out during the lavage procedure can implant leading to pregnancy which defeats the aim of PGD. Embryo recovery after superovulation seems to be more difficult than lavage following natural (mono) ovulation and fertilization (Winston, 1993).

Present day practice

Conventional IVF treatment has been the main method of generating embryos for PGD in contemporary practice although the couples may not necessarily be infertile. The only drawback of this method is that several spermatozoa normally become attached to the zona pellucida and these may later contaminate the biopsy microneedle thereby causing erroneous or conflicting results during genetic analysis, especially when polymerase chain reaction (PCR) is carried out. This consideration has now led to the use of ICSI for achieving fertilization of oocytes that are destined for PGD (Handyside, 1996).

Following genetic diagnosis, unaffected embryos are transferred back into the uterine cavity. The number of embryos to replace, following PGD, has been proposed at two. Apart from the avoidance of higher order multiple pregnancy this proposal aims at ensuring that access to individual fetuses, their amniotic fluid or placental tissue is not hampered by the presence of too many fetuses. The current strategy for PGD includes genetic diagnosis following conception to confirm that no genetically defective embryo was missed by PGD. Chorionic villus sampling or amniocentesis is required for obtaining fetal genetic material in these cases. However, not all centres restrict the number of transferred embryos thus.

Oocyte and embryo biopsy techniques

Initially, an opening has to be created in the zona pellucida to allow access to individual blastomeres for PGD. As has already been described in Chapters 9 and 14 this opening can be made by partial zona dissection (PZD), chemical zona drilling or the use of lasers. The timing of zona opening depends on the particular PGD

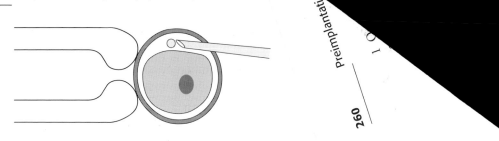

Figure 15.3 Polar body biopsy: a sharp microneedle pierces the zona pelluc the polar body.

approach that is to be used as described in the following sections. Polar body biopsy does not necessarily require opening of the zona; a glass micropipette is used to pierce the zona pellucida and aspirate the polar body.

Polar body biopsy

Polar body biopsy has been proposed as a method that will overcome some ethical and potential religious objections to PGD. Many religions that regard the embryo as the start of life do not accept PGD from the point of view that discarding the diseased embryos amounts to performing an abortion. The possibility of establishing genetic diagnosis at the oocyte stage before fertilization may assuage the concerns of some of these religious organizations or their members. The first polar body can be biopsied following oocyte retrieval. Prior to this, all cumulus cells are removed using hyaluronidase solution as described for ICSI in Chapter 9. This is to improve visualization of the oocyte structures and avoid contamination of the biopsy needle by extraneous DNA containing material. A micromanipulation set up similar to that of ICSI is used. The oocyte is positioned such that the first polar body is at 12 o'clock. It is then held in place by gentle suction using a blunt holding micropipette that is mounted on the left side. The sharp micropipette on the right side is used in piercing the zona pellucida and aspirating the first polar body which is then subjected to genetic analysis (Figure 15.3). The biopsied oocytes are inseminated 30–60 minutes later just as in conventional IVF treatment (Verlinsky & Kuliev, 1994). Selection of embryos for transfer will be from the group arising from oocytes that were shown through PGD not to be affected by the screened genetic disorder. Such diagnosis is possible by extrapolating findings made from genetic analysis of the first polar body. Montag et al. (1998) have recently described the use of laser microdissection to create a hole in the zona pellucida through which a blunt microneedle is introduced and used in aspirating the polar body.

The use of the first polar body for PGD suffers from quite a number of drawbacks that have been discussed by Handyside (1993), and Fasouliotis & Schenker (1998):

only maternal genetic defects can be screened.

2 Genetic diagnosis is indirect; inference on the genetic constitution of the oocyte itself is based on findings following genetic analysis of the first polar body. This may give erroneous results when there is genetic recombination during the (meiotic) cell division that gives rise to the first polar body.

3 The genetic status of the oocyte for the screened disease sometimes cannot be determined until genetic analysis of the second polar body is carried out. This means that the oocyte may have to be pierced twice with the biopsy microneedle and this may have associated deleterious effects on embryo viability. This will also lead to the same potential religious objections that PGD using the first polar body aims to avoid. The second polar body is extruded only at the time of fertilization, hence at the formation of new life, the embryo.

4 Polar body PGD cannot be used for the determination of transfer of autosomal dominant disease in the male.

5 Polar body PGD cannot be used for screening for the transfer of X-linked disease since the sex of the embryo cannot be determined by evaluation of the genetic material of only the oocyte.

6 It has been estimated that when screening for autosomal recessive diseases only 50% of the embryos will be available for embryo transfer because only the genetic composition of the oocyte is known. This contrasts with that of 75% of embryos following embryo biopsy and PGD, when the genetic contribution from the male is also known.

Blastomere biopsy

The genetic constitution of the embryo is established at the time of fertilization and derives from contributions from both the sperm and the oocyte nuclear material. Biopsy of the embryo will therefore allow optimal determination of the genetic make-up. PGD is preferably performed using two or more blastomeres to increase the accuracy of the results by allowing duplicate analysis. However, there is a limit to the number of blastomeres that can be removed from the early pre-implantation embryo without compromising its viability. Embryo biopsy is usually performed on the morning of the third day following oocyte retrieval when the embryo is expected to have 6–10 blastomeres. Genetic analysis is immediately carried out on these blastomeres and results should be available later that same day. This enables transfer of disease free embryos within 8–12 hours of the biopsy.

During the fertilization check that is normally carried out 18–22 hours following insemination of the retrieved oocytes, the cumulus cells are usually stripped away easily from their attachment to the zona pellucida. The micromanipulation set up is also used for blastomere biopsy. Following creation of the opening in the zona pellucida of the embryo a clean micro-pipette on the right side of the set-up

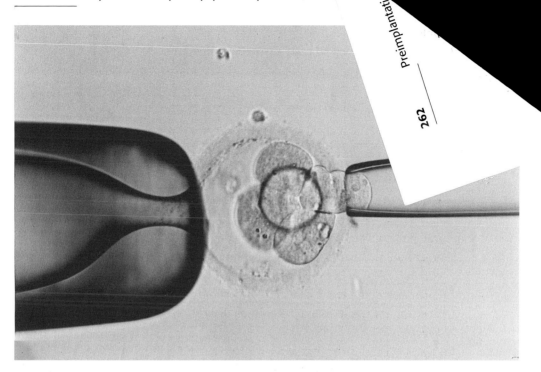

Figure 15.4 Biopsy of a cleavage stage embryo: after creating a hole in the zona pellucida the aspirating needle is introduced through the hole and used to aspirate one of the blastomeres. A second blastomere can be safely removed in 6–8 cell embryos.

is gently introduced through the hole and used in aspirating one or two blastomeres for analysis (Figure 15.4).

Blastocyst biopsy

Blastocyst formation usually occurs by the fifth day following ovulation (or oocyte retrieval). At that time the arrangement of cells within the embryo is seen to be in the form of an outer covering layer, called the trophectoderm, and an inner collection of cells at one pole of the embryo called the inner cell mass. The inner cell mass later forms the fetus proper while the trophectodermal cells form the placenta. Blastocyst biopsy aims at the removal of up to 10 trophectodermal cells for genetic analysis. PZD using the pipette rubbing method described in Chapter 14 is carried out at the pole of the blastocyst that is opposite to that of the inner cell mass to avoid inflicting any damage on the latter embryonic structure. Alternatively, this slit can be made using the laser (Veiga et al., 1997). After the slit is made in the zona pellucida the embryo is cultured overnight to allow expansion of the trophectodermal layer by fluid accumulation within the blastocyst cavity. This leads to herniation of part of the trophectoderm through the slit in the zona. The herniated cells are then excised with a microneedle (Figure 15.5) (Handyside, 1996) and subjected to genetic analysis.

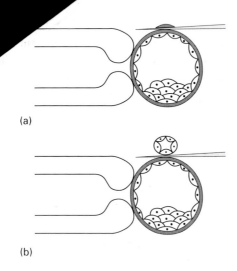

(a)

(b)

Figure 15.5 Blastocyst biopsy: (a) the zona pellucida is slit open away from the inner cell mass; and (b) after overnight culture, the herniated trophectoderm is excised with the microneedle.

Genetic analytical techniques for PGD

Only brief mention will be made of analytical techniques used for PGD. More details will be found in pioneer texts such as Fishel & Symmonds (1993), Fishel (1994), reports by the Hammersmith Hospital (London) group led by Handyside A. H. and Winston R. M. L., and the increasing scientific literature on PGD, some of which are listed in the bibliography.

The two main analytical techniques are fluorescence in situ hybridization (FISH) and PCR. FISH is carried out by first of all spreading the nuclei of the biopsied cell on a glass slide. Compounds that can react with components of specific chromosomes are then applied to the spread nuclei on the slide. Each of these compounds, also called chromosome-specific probes, is chemically attached to fluorescent compounds (i.e. fluorochrome-labelled). Following in situ hybridization the slide is visualized using specially equipped (fluorescent) microscopes. Each fluorochrome-labelled chromosome-specific probe produces a unique colour for the particular chromosome that it was designed to detect. There are now probes in several colours for the X and Y chromosomes and for an increasing number of the autosomes including chromosomes 1, 4, 6, 7, 13, 14, 15, 16, 17, 18, 21 and 22 (Bahce et al., 1999; Gianaroli et al., 1999). This makes it possible to test for the presence of many of these chromosomes and aneuploidies (abnormality of chromosome number) using just one blastomere.

PCR involves the repeated synthesis of a short segment of DNA within which the genetic anomaly that is being screened for resides. This DNA segment is derived from the nucleus of the embryonic cell that was removed from the embryo or the polar body from the oocyte. The amplification of the DNA fragment results in an exponential increase in the amount of genetic material such that it can be viewed by gel electrophoresis and staining. There are other and more complex PCR and FISH techniques which cannot be described in this book for example, fluorescent PCR.

Conclusion

PGD is still at its infancy but already many children (160 at the last estimate) have been born world-wide following this procedure which is now being carried out in 20 or more centres internationally (Fasouliotis & Schenker, 1998). There is no doubt that it is an important tool in the armamentarium of the geneticist. It is also closely tied with the development of assisted reproduction technology. There is hope that with further development of this technique a battery of specific gene and chromosome probes will become available for screening embryos generated by older women. This is to enable identification of abnormal embryos which are believed to be more prevalent in these women; transfer of only healthy embryos may result in better pregnancy rates and outcome. There are a number of problems to overcome before this becomes feasible not least of which is the poor follicular development and oocyte recovery commonly found in these women.

Specially formulated embryo culture media are now being used in an attempt to successfully grow more embryos in the laboratory until the blastocyst stage before transfer into the uterus. This allows more opportunity to detect the best growing embryos such that their uterine transfer will improve conception rates following routine IVF treatment. This current move may impact on the practice of PGD. For example, more time could be allowed for genetic analysis following cleavage stage embryo biopsy; embryo transfer is safely deferred to 24 or 48 hours after the biopsy. Alternatively, embryo biopsy can be routinely delayed until the blastocyst stage so that more cells could be biopsied. However, blastocyst transfer is not yet routinely carried out for all patients and there are still a number of unresolved issues such as what to do about the significant number of women whose embryos do not develop into blastocysts during in vitro culture.

BIBLIOGRAPHY

Ao, A., Wells, D., Handyside, A. H. et al. (1998). Preimplantation genetic diagnosis of inherited cancer: familial adenomatous polyposis coli. *Journal of Assisted Reproduction and Genetics* **15**, 140–4.

Avner, R., Reubinoff, B. E., Simon, A. et al. (1996). Management of rhesus isoimmunization by preimplantation genetic diagnosis. *Molecular Human Reproduction* 2, 60–2.

Bahce, M., Cohen, J. & Munne, S. (1999). Preimplantation genetic diagnosis of aneuploidy: were we looking at the wrong chromosomes? *Journal of Assisted Reproduction and Genetics* 16, 176–81.

Fasouliotis, S. J. & Schenker, J. G. (1998). Preimplantation genetic diagnosis principles and ethics. *Human Reproduction* 13, 2238–45.

Fishel, S. (Ed.) (1994). *Micromanipulation Techniques. Bailliere's Clinical Obstetrics and Gynaecology*, 8.

Fishel, S. & Symmonds, M. (Eds) (1993). *Gamete and Embryo Micromanipulation in Human Reproduction*. London: Edward Arnold Publishers.

Gianaroli, L., Magli, M. C., Ferraretti, A. P. et al. (1997). Preimplantation genetic diagnosis increases the implantation rate in human in vitro fertilization by avoiding the transfer of chromosomally abnormal embryos. *Fertility and Sterility* 68, 1128–31.

Gianaroli, L., Magli, M. C., Munne, S. et al. (1999). Advantages of day 4 embryo transfer in patients undergoing preimplantation genetic diagnosis of aneuploidy. *Journal of Assisted Reproduction and Genetics* 16, 170–5.

Handyside, A. H. (1993). Pre-implantation diagnosis: strategies for embryo biopsy and genetic analysis. In *Gamete and Embryo Micromanipulation in Human Reproduction*, ed. S. Fishel & M. Symmonds, pp. 173–82. London: Edward Arnold Publishers.

Handyside, A. H. (1996). Preimplantation genetic diagnosis today. In *Human Conception In Vitro, 1995*, ed. H. W. Jones, Jnr., J. Cohen & L. Hamberger, *Human Reproduction* 11 (Suppl.1), 139–55.

Kilpatrick, M. W., Harton, G. L., Phylactou, L. A. et al. (1996). Preimplantation genetic diagnosis in Marfan syndrome. *Fetal Diagnosis and Therapy* 11, 402–6.

Lee, S. H., Kwak, I. P., Cha, K. E. et al. (1998). Preimplantation diagnosis of non-deletion Duchenne muscular dystrophy (DMD) by linkage polymerase chain reaction analysis. *Molecular Human Reproduction* 4, 345–9.

Lissens, W., Sermon, K., Staessen, C. et al. (1996). Review: preimplantation diagnosis of inherited disease. *Journal of Inherited Metabolic Disease* 19, 709–23.

Montag, M., van der Ven, K., Delacretaz, G. et al. (1998). Laser-assisted microdissection of the zona pellucida facilitates polar body biopsy. *Fertility and Sterility* 69, 539–42.

Munne, S. & Weier, H. U. (1996). Simultaneous enumeration of chromosomes 13, 18, 21, X, and Y in interphase cells for preimplantation genetic diagnosis of aneuploidy. *Cytogenetics and Cell Genetics* 75, 263–7.

Rechitsky, S., Strom, C., Verlinsky, O. et al. (1999). Accuracy of preimplantation diagnosis of single-gene disorders by polar body analysis of oocytes. *Journal of Assisted Reproduction and Genetics* 16, 192–8.

Reubinoff, B. E., Lewin, A., Verner, M. et al. (1997). Intracytoplasmic sperm injection combined with preimplantation genetic diagnosis for the prevention of recurrent gestational trophoblastic disease. *Human Reproduction* 12, 805–8.

Snowdon, C. & Green, J. M. (1997). Preimplantation diagnosis and other reproductive options: attitudes of male and female carriers of recessive disorders. *Human Reproduction* 12, 341–50.

Soussis, I., Harper, J. C., Handyside, A. H. & Winston, R. M. (1996). Obstetric outcome of pregnancies resulting from embryos biopsied for pre-implantation diagnosis of inherited disease. *British Journal of Obstetrics and Gynaecology* **103**, 784–8.

Staessen, C., van Assche, E., Joris, H. et al. (1999). Clinical experience of sex determination by fluorescent in-situ hybridization for preimplantation genetic diagnosis. *Molecular Human Reproduction* **5**, 382–9.

Veiga, A., Sandalinas, M., Benkhalifa, M. et al. (1997). Laser blastocyst biopsy for preimplantation diagnosis in the human. *Zygote* **5**, 351–4.

Verlinsky, Y. & Kuliev, A. (1994). Human preimplantation diagnosis: needs, efficiency and efficacy of genetic and chromosomal analysis. In *Micromanipulation Techniques*, ed. S. Fishel, *Bailliere's Clinical Obstetrics and Gynaecology* **8**, 177–96.

Verlinsky, Y., Rechitsky, S., Cieslak, J. et al. (1997). Preimplantation diagnosis of single gene disorders by two-step oocyte genetic analysis using first and second polar body. *Biochemical and Molecular Medicine* **62**, 182–7.

Winston, R. M. L. (1993). An overview of pre-implantation diagnosis. In *Gamete and Embryo Micromanipulation in Human Reproduction*, ed. S. Fishel & M. Symmonds, pp. 165–72. London: Edward Arnold Publishers.

Xu, K., Shi, Z. M., Veeck, L. L. et al. (1999). First unaffected pregnancy using preimplantation genetic diagnosis for sickle cell anaemia. *Journal of the American Medical Association* **281**, 1701–6.

Appendix

ACRONYMS IN ASSISTED REPRODUCTION TECHNOLOGY

There is a continually expanding list of acronyms that represent different techniques that can be applied during assisted conception treatment of infertile couples. Others relate to investigations, medical and surgical treatments, and the names of disease conditions. It is important that the reader is informed on their meaning because many sound rather trendy and will be used preferentially by professionals working in this area. Competition for international usage has been fierce with some not quite making the grade. Every pioneer and inventor in this area seems to have something they wish to be included in such lists.

Acronym	Meaning
AIH	Artificial insemination (with) husband (sperm)
ART	Assisted reproduction technology
ASA	Antisperm antibodies
AZF	Azoospermia factor
BBT	Basal body temperature (monitoring)
BSO	Bilateral salpingo-oophorectomy
CASA	Computer assisted semen analysis
CBAVD	Congenital bilateral absence of the vas deferens
CC	Clomiphene citrate
CISS	Computer image sperm selection
COH	Controlled ovarian hyperstimulation
D&C	Dilatation and curettage
DI	Donor insemination (used to be called AID, artificial insemination donor, until the advent of AIDS)
DIFI	Direct intrafollicular insemination
DIPI	Direct intraperitoneal insemination
DNA	Deoxyribonucleic acid
DOT	Direct oocyte transfer
E1	Oestrone
E2	Oestradiol
E3	Oestriol
ELISA	Enzyme-linked immunoadsorption assay
ELSI	Elongated spermatid injection

Acronym	Meaning
ERPC	Evacuation of retained products of conception
ET	Embryo transfer
FER	Frozen embryo replacement
FET	Frozen embryo transfer
FISH	Fluorescent in situ hybridization
FREDI	Fallopian replacement of eggs with delayed insemination
FSH	Follicle stimulating hormone
GIFT	Gamete intrafallopian transfer
GIPT	Gametes intraperitoneal transfer
GnRH	Gonadotrophin releasing hormone
GnRHa	Gonadotrophin releasing hormone analogue (or agonist)
GV	Germinal vesicle (oocyte)
hCG	Human chorionic gonadotrophin
HIC-IVF	High insemination concentration in vitro fertilization
hMG	Human menopausal gonadotrophin
HOST	Hypo-osmotic swelling test
HPF	High power field
HRT	Hormone replacement therapy
HSA	Human serum albumin
HSG	Hysterosalpingogram, hysterosalpingograph, hysterosalpingography
IBT	Immunobead test
ICI	Intracervical insemination
ICM	Inner cell mass
ICSI	Intracytoplasmic sperm injection
IPI	Intraperitoneal insemination
ITI	Intratubal insemination
IUCD	Intrauterine contraceptive device
IUI	Intrauterine insemination
IVC	Intravaginal culture
IVF	In vitro fertilization
Lap & Dye	Laparoscopy and dye test
LH	Luteinizing hormone
MAF	Microassisted fertilization
MAR test	Mixed antiglobulin reaction test (for detecting seminal ASA!)
MESA	Microepididymal sperm aspiration
MFT	Male fertility test (semen analysis)
μIVF	Microdrop in vitro fertilization
MSU	Mid-stream urine
OAT	Oligoasthenoteratozoospermia
OC	Oral contraceptive
OCC	Oocyte cumulus complex
OD	Oocyte donation (oocyte donor)
OPU	Ovum pick-up
OR	Oocyte recipient
P	Progesterone

Acronym	Meaning
PCO	Polycystic ovaries
PCOD	Polycystic ovary disease
PCOS	Polycystic ovary syndrome
PCR	Polymerase chain reaction
PCT	Post coital test
PESA	Percutaneous epididymal sperm aspiration
PGD	Pre-implantation genetic diagnosis
PID	Pelvic inflammatory disease
POD	Pouch of Douglas
POF	Premature ovarian failure
POST	Peritoneal oocyte and sperm transfer
ProST	Pronuclear stage transfer
PZD	Partial zona dissection
ROS	Reactive oxygen species
ROSI	Round spermatid injection
ROSNI	Microinjection of round spermatid nuclei into oocytes
SA	Semen analysis
SCI	Spinal cord injured (patient)
SCMC	Sperm-cervical-mucus-contact (test)
SET	Surgical embryo transfer
SPA	Sperm penetration assay
STD	Sexually transmitted disease
SUZI	Subzonal insemination
T3	Tri-iodothyronine
T4	Thyroxine
TAH	Total abdominal hysterectomy
TAT	Tray agglutination test (for detecting ASA)
TESA	Testicular sperm aspiration
TESE	Testicular sperm extraction
TEST	Tubal embryo stage transfer
TET	Tubal embryo transfer
TSET	Transfer of sperms and eggs to tubes
TSH	Thyroid stimulating hormone
TUFT	Transuterine fallopian transfer
UFO	Unfertilized oocyte
VITI	Vaginal intratubal transfer
ZD	Zona drilling
ZIFT	Zygote intrafallopian transfer
ZPD	Zona pellucida drilling

Index